Medical Evidence in Veterans' Disability Rating

David Anaise, M.D., J.D.
Sharon Anaise-Benham, M.D.

Medical Evidence in Veterans' Disability Rating

Copyright © 2016 by
David Anaise, M.D., J.D.
Sharon Anaise-Benham, M.D.
All rights reserved.

No part of this publication may be reproduced in whole or in part, or stored in a retrieval system, or transmitted in any form or by any means, electronic, mechanical, photocopying, recording, or otherwise, without written permission of the author.

Printed in the United States of America
University of Arizona Libraries
Express Document Center
Tucson, Arizona

ISBN 1542726581 ISBN 13 is 9781542726580;

Table of Contents

CHAPTER 1: Managing a Veteran's Disability 1
    Claim 2
    The VA Disability Rating System 2
    The VA Disability Adjudication System 5
    The VA Disability Benefits Rating Table 9

CHAPTER 2: Independent Medical Opinion (IMO) and Nexus Letters for Disabled Veterans 17
    What is a Nexus? 17
    What is an Independent Medical Opinion (IMO)? 17
    Why Do Veterans Need an IMO/ Nexus Letter? 18
    Requirements for an Adequate Medical Opinion – Why is a Veteran's Primary Physician's Opinion Often Insufficient? .. 19
    The Importance of Published Medical Reports (Treatises) in an IMO 23
    BVA Decision Held that Obstructive Sleep Apnea (OSA) is Secondary to Posttraumatic Stress Disorder (PTSD) Based on this Author's IMO 25
    BVA Decision Held that OSA is Secondary to Asthma Based on this Author's IMO 26

CHAPTER 3: Total Disability Based On Individual Unemployability (TDIU) 27
    TDIU Requires that a Veteran Be Unable to Secure Substantially Gainful Occupation 27
    Individual Unemployability – Consideration of Educational and Occupational History 30
    What is the Effective Date for TDIU? 31
    Is VA Form 21-8940 "Veteran's Application for Increased Compensation Based on Unemployability" Mandatory in a TDIU claim? 35
    What is the Effect of a Favorable Social Security Disability Decision on a Veteran's Disability Claim? 36

CHAPTER 4: Sleep Apnea 39

    Service-connected Conditions That Cause
Obstructive Sleep Apnea (OSA) 39
What is Obstructive Sleep Apnea? 41
Rating for Sleep Apnea.. 43
Development of Sleep Apnea During Military
Service.. 45
Sleep Apnea Secondary to Service-Connected Sinusitis,
Rhinitis or Deviated Septum 47
Sleep Apnea Secondary to Service-Connected PTSD.............. 50
Sleep Apnea Secondary to Chronic Pain Syndrome................ 56
Sleep Apnea Secondary to Narcotics Prescribed
for Service-Connected Conditions 59
Sleep Apnea Secondary to Service-Connected
Tinnitus 60
Sleep Apnea Secondary to Service-Connected
Chronic Obstructive Airway Disease (COPD) or
Asthma 63
Sleep Apnea Secondary to Service-Connected
Gastroesophageal Reflux Disease (GERD) 66
Sleep Apnea and Obesity... 68
Sleep Apnea Secondary to Service-Connected
Diabetes Mellitus 70
Sleep Apnea Secondary to Service-Connected Stroke
and Ischemic Heart Disease 71
Sleep Apnea Secondary to Service-Connected
Cervical Spine Abnormalities 72
Migraines Secondary to Service-Connected
Sleep Apnea.. 75
Hypertension Secondary to Service-Connected
Sleep Apnea.. 75

    Sleep Apnea Secondary to Service-Connected Fibromyalgia . 76
Upper Airway Resistance Syndrome (UARS) 77
Sleep Apnea Caused by Antidepressants 78
Narcolepsy.. 80
Sleep Apnea and Interstitial Lung Disease 81

Sleep Apnea and Cardiovascular Disease (CVD) 83
Sleep Apnea and Headaches/Migraines.. 85

CHAPTER 5: Orthopedics 87

Posttraumatic Osteoarthritis 87
The BVA Accepted This Author's IMO Regarding
Osteoarthritis 92
Understanding the Rating of Knee Injury 93
    Knee Anatomy 94
    Knee Conditions 94
    Limitation of Motion.. 97
Evaluation of Pain 102
How is the Functional Assessment of Joints
Conducted? 104
Combined Rating and the Rule Against
Pyramiding 106
Proposed Amendment to the Rating of
Musculoskeletal Conditions 109
Understanding the New Rating Table for Cervical
and Lumbar Spine Disability 113
What is Intervertebral Disc Syndrome (IVDS)? 115
    The pertinent anatomy for IVDS.. 115
    Cause of IVDS 117
    Symptoms of IVDS 117
    Diagnosis of IVDS 119
    Treatment of IVDS 120
    Rating for IVDS.. 122
    Incapacitating Episodes 124
What Does a VA Examiner Look for in
Musculoskeletal Rating? 126
Signs Suggesting that a Veteran is Malingering
or Exaggerating His Symptoms 127
Degenerative Joint Disease Rating Based on
Objective Tests.. 129
    Sciatic Nerve Function... 129
    Common Peroneal Nerve Function 130

How do the New Evaluation Criteria for IVDS
Compare to the Old Criteria? 131
       Over evaluations 132
Neuropathy 132
Ankle injury in paratroopers - Tarsal Tunnel
Syndrome 136
Rating for Shoulder Disability 137

CHAPTER 6: Cardiology 141

Atherosclerosis and Coronary Risk Factors 141
Elevated Cholesterol Levels During Service
Leads to Coronary Artery Disease 142
Rating of Coronary Artery Disease 143
The Value of Stress Testing 145
Stress Testing and METS 145

CHAPTER 7: Gastrointestinal System 155

Irritable Bowel Syndrome (IBS) Secondary
to Service-Connected Posttraumatic Stress
Disorder (PTSD) 155
Crohn's Disease 158
       Establishing the Diagnosis of Crohn's
       Disease and Evaluating Disease Activity 159
       Stress Can be a Contributing Factor in
       Crohn's Disease 160
       Fatty Liver 161
Gastroesophageal Reflux Disease (GERD) 163

CHAPTER 8: Neurology 166

Traumatic Brain Injury (TBI) 166
       Brain Injury Severity 169
       TBI Residuals 171
Posttraumatic Headaches 173

Tinnitus 175

CHAPTER 9: Rheumatology 179

Chronic Fatigue Syndrome and Fibromyalgia 179
Systemic Lupus Erythematosus 188
    Antinuclear Antibody Test 189
Rheumatoid Arthritis 193
    Pathogenesis of Rheumatoid Arthritis 195
    Clinical Features of Rheumatoid Arthritis 196
    Constitutional Features of Rheumatoid
    Arthritis 197
    Carpal Tunnel Syndrome in Rheumatoid
    Arthritis 197

CHAPTER 10: Endocrinology 198

Diabetes Mellitus - Etiology and Classification 198
    Diagnosis of Diabetes Mellitus 199
    BVA Decision Regarding Service
    Connection for Diabetes Mellitus 202
    Inhaled Corticosteroids and the Risk of
    Diabetes Onset and Progression 204
    Diabetes and Renal Failure 204
    Hypertension and Diabetes Mellitus 206
    Diabetic Cataracts 207
    Prostatic Hypertrophy and Diabetes
    Mellitus 208

CHAPTER 11: Psychiatry 210

Winning a Claim for Posttraumatic Stress
Disorder (PTSD) Benefits 210
What Did the VA PTSD Study Find? 211
What is Posttraumatic Stress Disorder (PTSD)? 213

Does a Veteran Need to Prove That He/She
Was Involved in Combat for a PTSD Claim............................ 215
What Evidence is Required to Prove Combat
Stressors? 220
What Evidence is Required to Prove a Personal or
Sexual Assault? 222
Is the Veteran's Own Testimony Sufficient to
Establish a Stressor? 224
Alcohol and Drug Abuse in PTSD Cases................................ 225
Psychological Testing in PTSD Claims.................................. 226
Rating Considerations for PTSD 228
Hypertension Secondary to PTSD.. 232

CHAPTER 12: Toxicology 237

Agent Orange 237
Oral Cancer Caused by Exposure to Agent Orange................ 240
Myelodysplastic Syndrome (MDS) Due to
Exposure to Agent Orange 244
Hypertension, Vascular Disease and Chronic
Respiratory Diseases Due to Exposure to
Agent Orange 247
Bladder Cancer Due to Exposure to Agent Orange 248
Prostate Cancer and Trichloroethylene (TCE)
Exposure 251
Parkinson Disease and Trichloroethylene (TCE)
Exposure 254
Camp Lejeune 255
Gulf War Syndrome 259

CHAPTER 13: Erectile Dysfunction 264

Erectile Dysfunction Secondary to Hypertension 267
Erectile Dysfunction Secondary to Sleep Apnea.................... 268
Erectile Dysfunction Secondary to PTSD 268
Diabetes is an Established Risk Factor for

Sexual Dysfunction 270

CHAPTER 14: Claims for Disability Due to VA Negligent Care Pursuant to U.S.C.S. 1151 272

CHAPTER 15: Proposed Reduction in VA Benefits.. 277

APPENDIX A: CV David Anaise M.D., J.D 284

INTRODUCTION

This book is intended to help Veteran Service Organization representatives better pursue the complex medical and legal issues involved in establishing veteran disability rating. I also hope that this book will stimulate a discussion to bring the antiquated rating table into the 21st century.

Recent statistics show that the Board of Veterans' Appeals (BVA) only approves 17% to 28% of cases. Fortunately, the U.S. Court of Appeals for Veterans' Claims (CAVC) reverses the majority of the adverse BVA decisions. Between 1995-2006, the CAVC heard 18,000 cases in which veterans had been denied benefits at the BVA level. In almost 80% of the cases, the CAVC either reversed the BVA decision or remanded the case for re-adjudication. These statistics demonstrate the need for improved claim processing that will allow for correct rating at the initial review.

I am an attorney specializing in disability law and also a Board-Certified surgeon (transplant surgery) still licensed to practice medicine. As my curriculum vitae indicates [Appendix A], I am a surgeon with almost thirty years of medical experience. I was Clinical Associate Professor of Surgery and Attending Surgeon in Transplantation at SUNY at Stony Brook. I served as President of the New York Transplantation Society and as Assistant Editor of Transplantation Proceedings. I hold three patents. I have authored three book chapters and 106 research papers published in peer reviewed medical journals. I am also most proud of being a combat veteran. In 1973, I served in the Israeli Seventh Brigade (armored) during the Yom Kippur war.

After representing more than 3,000 claimants before the Social Security Administration (SSA) and winning numerous appeals at the Federal Court, I have restricted my practice to the representation of veterans. I am passionate about defending veterans' rights and firmly believe that my medical career gives me a great advantage in understanding and challenging faulty medical rating decisions. As an attorney admitted to practice before the U.S. Court of Appeals for Veterans Claims, I am committed to understanding the very complex legal rules and decisions involved.

CASES LITIGATED BEFORE THE CAVC

MU v. Shinseki 09-3570
RK v. Shinseki 13-2908
EW v. Shinseki 12-2155
HH v. Shinseki 11-1612
RCR v. McDonald 15-760
LCW v. McDonald 15-2697
JH v. McDonald 16-1515

Law offices of David Anaise MD
1001 W San Martin Dr.
Tucson AZ 85704
520-219-7321
520-219-7344
Fax 520-844-1452
anaisedavid.office@gmail.com

DEDICATION

This book is dedicated to the veterans of the Seventh Brigade with whom I served as a captain of the Medical Corps during the Yom Kippur War.

On October 6, 1973, the Syrian 7th Infantry Division attacked the Israeli 7th Armored Brigade, comprised of only two tank battalions, in the Golan Heights. The Syrians launched simultaneous attacks from the north and from the south. They attacked the two Israeli brigades and eleven supporting artillery batteries with five divisions (the 7th, 9th and 5th, with the 1st and 3rd in reserve) and 188 batteries.

The Syrians began their attack with an airstrike of about 100 aircrafts and a 50-minute artillery barrage. At the start of the battle, approximately 400 of the Syrian tanks were T-62s, the most modern Soviet-bloc tank at the time. The Syrian plan called for its 5th, 7th and 9th mechanized infantry divisions, in BTR-50 armored personnel carriers (APCs) supported by 900 tanks, to breach the Israeli lines, opening the way for the 1st and 3rd armored divisions to move in with their 500 tanks to capture the entire Golan Heights before Israel had a chance to mobilize. Initially, Israel was able to deploy only 176 tanks.

The Syrians started the offensive. Mine-clearing tanks and bridge-layers led the way to overcome the Israeli obstacles. The Syrians gained much ground at the start, but failed to move tanks across the anti-tank ditch.

They penetrated the Israeli defenses at night with the help of night vision equipment—equipment that the Israelis lacked.

The next day, the Syrians mounted a second attack. At one point in the engagement less than forty Israeli tanks were facing approximately 500 Syrian tanks; the Barak Brigade had only 15 serviceable tanks.

Every Israeli tank deployed on the Golan Heights was engaged during the initial attacks. Reservists were alerted and quickly began to arrive at the scene. Immediately upon arriving at army depots the reservists were sent directly to the front lines; they did not have time to wait for the crews they trained with, machine guns to be installed on the tanks, or even calibrate the tank guns (a time-consuming process known as bore-sighting). The Syrians expected that it would take at least 24 hours for Israeli reserves to reach the front lines. Reserve units began reaching the battle lines only 15 hours after the war began. Israeli reserve forces approaching the Golan Heights were subjected to Syrian artillery fire directed from Mount Hermon.

On the second and third day, Syrian forces suffered heavy losses as Israeli tanks and infantry fought desperately to buy time for all the reserve forces to reach the front lines. Stopgap blocking actions were conducted whenever the Syrians were on the verge of breaking through. However, in spite of their losses, the Syrians continued to press the attack. The vastly outnumbered Israeli defenses lost numerous tanks. By the afternoon of October 9th, the 7th Brigade was down to six tanks protecting what was for all intents and purposes a clear path into Israel's north.

On the fourth day, the 7th Brigade received a small reinforcement force; it now had less than a dozen operating tanks and was almost out of ammunition. The Syrians, exhausted from three days of continuous fighting and unaware of how close to victory they actually were, turned in retreat. Hundreds of destroyed tanks and APCs littering the valley below the Israeli ramparts were testimony to the horrible destruction that had taken place there. Within 5 days, the Syrians had lost almost 1,000 tanks. The Syrians retreated for reasons that are still debated.

(http://en.wikipedia.org/wiki/Valley_of_Tears)

CHAPTER 1 - MANAGING A VETERAN'S DISABILITY CLAIM

The VA Disability Rating System

Unlike the Social Security Administration (SSA), which grants benefits to individuals who are unable to work at any job in the national economy, the Veterans' Administration (VA) grants benefits to veterans whose disabilities can decrease their potential ability to earn a living. The VA rating system evaluates a veteran's disability by degrees of impairment from 0-100%, in increments of 10%. The lowest compensable rating is 10%, which provides for monthly benefits of $115 (as of December, of 2006). A 100% rating provides for a monthly compensation of $2,471.

The VA provides a detailed disability rating table, which is broken down into sections pertaining to various organs or classes of diseases. Each body system contains a series of diagnoses, each with a numerical diagnostic code. Each diagnosis is then broken down into levels of disability ratings ranging from 0-100%.

As the severity of disease symptomatology increases so does the disability rating. For example, a rating of 30% for ulcerative colitis connotes moderately severe colitis with frequent exacerbations, whereas a rating of 100% for ulcerative colitis requires symptoms of pronounced colitis with marked malnutrition, anemia, and general debility.

Even obtaining a rating of 0% for a condition is important, in that it sets the ground for increasing the rating at a later time if the condition gets worse, without the need to prove service connection.

Analogous ratings are provided for disabilities that are not listed in the rating schedule but that could be rated under a closely related disease or injury.

The Schedule for Rating Disabilities is comprised of ten grades representing the effect a disability has on the veteran's earning capacity. As the following table shows, the compensation to veterans with increasing disability grades is not linear – a veteran with a 90% disability rating could almost double his award by adding an additional 10% to his rating.

VA Disability Compensation Rates for Veterans (2011)	
Veteran's Disability Rating	Monthly Rate Paid to Veterans
10 %	$123
20 %	$243
30 %	$376
40 %	$541
50 %	$770
60 %	$974
70 %	$1,228
80 %	$1,427
90 %	$1,604
100 %	$2,673

A rating of 100% means a veteran is totally disabled. It is very rare for an injury to one organ or limb to amount to a rating of 100%. Most veterans with a 100% rating have injuries to two or more organs or limbs.

Multiple disability ratings for various organs and limbs, however, are not simply added to reach a total disability grade. If there are two or more service-connected disabilities, the overall percentage is computed by "combining" the individual ratings, not by adding them together. For example, a 30% service-connected rating for one condition, plus a 20% service-connected rating for another condition, will result in a 40% combined rating, not 50%.

The VA uses a complex combination formula that considers how additional disability ratings impact a veteran's already disabled state, rather than considering how multiple disability ratings would impact a non-disabled person. Consider, for example, a veteran with a 60% disability rating for one organ and a 30% disability rating for another organ. As mentioned above, the veteran does not simply have a cumulative disability rating of 90%. Instead, the VA looks at the veteran's most disabling condition, the 60% rating, and considers the veteran to be a 40% efficient person. The next disability rating, 30%, is then considered in light of this 40 % efficiency, and the veteran is now considered to lose 30% of his remaining 40% efficiency, which is 12%. This means the veteran is now considered only 28% efficient, which leaves the veteran with a disability rating of 72% (rounded down to 70% under VA rules).

The rating system is published in a schedule (38 C.F.R. § 4.25) that allows rating officials to quickly determine combined ratings. This formula ensures that combined ratings for multiple organs will never reach a full 100%, making it almost impossible for veterans with multiple disability ratings to reach 100%.

The VA, however, has recognized that this rating system often fails to reflect the combined effect of the veteran's multiple injuries on his ability to work. If a veteran cannot achieve a 100% disability rating under the system detailed above, the VA may assign a total disability rating (100%) if the VA determines that the veteran is unable to secure a substantially gainful occupation. 38 C.F.R. § 4.16.

Total Disability Individual Unemployability (TDIU) ratings consider the effect that combined service-connected disabilities have on a particular veteran's ability to work. An award of TDIU is based on an acknowledgement that even though an objectively correct rating under the ratings schedule produces a disability rating of less than 100%, subjective factors may permit assigning a 100% disability rating to the particular veteran under particular facts (*Norris v. West*, 12 Vet. App. 413, 1999). TDIU determination is considered in the context of an individual veteran's specific vocational capabilities, regardless of whether an average person would be rendered unemployable under similar circumstances (*Hattlestad (II) v. Derwinski*, 3 Vet. App. 213 (1992)). See also VA Gen. Prec. 75-91 (Dec. 27, 1991).

The VA Disability Adjudication System

The vast majority of Veterans' claims for disability are denied. Once a claim is denied, a Notice of Disagreement (NOD) must be filed within one year of the rating decision. A few months after an NOD is filed, the regional office (RO) will send the veteran an Appeals Election Form asking the veteran to select between the Traditional Appeals Process and the Decision Review Officer (DRO).

The DRO is a senior officer at the regional office who will review the case and has the power to award benefits. Prior to the DRO making any decision in a case, he/she will either offer the veteran a hearing or ask the veteran whether there is any additional information to provide.

Once the DRO makes a decision, that decision is issued to the veteran in a Statement of the Case (SOC). In order to appeal this decision, the rules require that a Form 9, Appeal to the Board of Veterans' Appeals, be filed within 60 days from the date of the SOC.

Once the Form 9 is submitted to the VA, the case waits until the RO certifies it to the BVA. The BVA is poorly staffed, thus, cases are slowly trickled to the BVA from the RO. It takes approximately 3 to 5 years from when a Form 9 is filed for a case to be heard by the BVA.

A claim follows a different track depending on which type of BVA hearing is selected on the Form 9. If the veteran waives the hearing, the case is prepared for transfer to the BVA and no further development occurs at the RO level. The RO prepares a VA Form 8,

Certification of Appeal, which indicates that the case is being transferred to the BVA. Once the case is docketed at the BVA, the veteran is sent a letter informing him/her that he/she has 90 days to submit additional evidence or argument.

Many veterans defeat this fast track by submitting additional claims or evidence to the RO. The case, then, instead of progressing to the BVA, ends up lingering at the RO for additional development and the issuance of a Supplemental Statement of the Case (SSOC).

If a veteran requests a BVA Travel Board hearing on the Form 9, the RO typically sends a letter to the veteran acknowledging the request for a hearing, but also attempting to persuade the veteran to request a different mode of BVA review. The letter explains that it could be months or years until a Travel Board hearing is scheduled, owing to the backlog of requests and the infrequency of the hearings. The letter advises the veteran that he/she may choose to remain on the waiting list for a Travel Board hearing.

In 2009, the wait time for a hearing was 771 days. The average length of time between filing the Form 9 and the Board's disposition was **886 days**. Veterans can definitely shave off two years of waiting by waiving the hearing and asking the BVA to rule based on a written appeal.

Source: Annual Report of the Chairman, Board of Veterans' Appeals, Fiscal Year 2010, p. 19.

http://www.bva.va.gov/docs/Chairmans_Annual_Rpts/BVA2010AR.pdf

	Responsible Party	**Average Elapsed Time Interval Processing Time**
Notice of Disagreement Receipt to Statement of the Case	Regional Office	243 days
Statement of the Case Issuance to Substantive Appeal Receipt	Claimant	42 days
Substantive Appeal Receipt to Certification of Appeal to BVA	Regional Office	609 days
Receipt of Certified Appeal to Issuance of BVA Decision	BVA	212 days
Average Remand Time Factor	Regional Office	493 days

In 2009, the following wait times existed in cases in which hearings were requested:

	Type of Hearing	Average Elapsed Time Interval
Substantive Appeal Receipt to Date of Hearing	Travel Board	743 days
Substantive Appeal Receipt to Date of Hearing	Videoconference	678 days
Substantive Appeal Receipt to Date of Hearing	Central Office (DC)	771 days

There are certain things a veteran can do to expedite his/her case:

1. The veteran should not assume that his/her claim file contains current medical records. The veteran is advised to go to his/her local VA and obtain a copy of the last two years of his/her medical records and provide these records to his/her representative.

2. The veteran should write a short narrative describing the major issues on appeal and what evidence there is that they occurred while in service.

3. The veteran should significantly limit the number of claims made. This is especially true if a

veteran already has service-connected disabilities with a combined rating above 80%. To get from 80% to 90% the veteran requires an additional disability of 50%. An additional disability of 10% will grant only 2%, and this will roll back the combined disability rating to 80% (*See "The VA Disability Rating System"*). The VA, rather than dealing with the conditions that are best detailed and are likely to grant a veteran the highest percentage of disability, will move to resolve the additional small claims by scheduling additional examinations. This alone may delay the case by 2 to 3 years.

The VA Disability Benefits Rating Table

The VA Disability Benefits Program is unique among other disability programs. Other disability programs, such as the Social Security Administration or long-term disability insurance companies, pay the insured only when he is unable to either work at his regular job (LTD) or if he is unable to work at any job in the national economy (SSA).

The VA pays a veteran if he/she suffered injuries that in theory will reduce his/her potential for earning. The veteran does not have to prove that he/she is unable to perform his/her job. The veteran merely needs to show that his/her medical condition meets the diagnosis and description of degree of severity in the VA's Schedule for Rating Disabilities (hereafter referred to as the Rating Schedule).

Title 38, United States Code, Section 355 provides for the adoption of a Schedule for Rating Disabilities by the VA. This schedule serves as the official guide for classifying clinical findings and converting these findings into degrees of disability.

The Rating Schedule is a guide for evaluating disability resulting from all types of diseases and injuries sustained while serving in the military service. The disease or injury need not be the result of combat action.

In December of 1988, the General Accounting Office (GAO) reviewed the medical criteria the VA used in its Rating Schedule to determine whether the Rating Schedule reflected current medical advances and terminology to enable rating specialists to make accurate and uniform disability decisions. The GAO found:

1. The VA has periodically revised parts of the Rating Schedule, but has not comprehensively revised the Schedule since 1945 and has not revised 10 of 14 Schedule sections since 1978;

2. The VA lacked a systematic process for reviewing Schedule sections;

3. The VA, military, and private physicians reviewing the Schedule identified examples of outdated terminology, poorly defined impairments, and common medical conditions missing from the Schedule;

4. The VA rating specialists cited concerns about their ability to accurately and uniformly rate

disabilities with the Schedule, since it used diagnostic codes, which did not distinguish between degrees of severity and did not list all medical conditions identified in medical examination reports.

Since early colonial days, various methods of rating disabilities have been used to award veterans benefits. The War Risk Insurance Act of 1917 created a rating schedule and provided the framework for today's Compensation and Pension programs for disabled veterans. The Schedule was revised in 1921, 1925, 1933, and 1945; the 1945 Rating Schedule serves as the basis for current disability decisions.

Federal law (38 U.S.C. 355) states that the VA Administrator shall "adopt and apply a schedule of ratings of reductions in earning capacity from specific injuries or combination of injuries. The ratings shall be based, as far as practicable, upon the average impairments of earning capacity resulting from such injuries in civil occupations."

The current Rating Schedule, developed in 1945, was published in 1946. It contains 14 sections; 1 has not been revised since 1964 and only 4 have been revised since 1978. Even the four sections of the Rating Schedule that the VA revised since 1978 do not represent a comprehensive update of medical criteria.

Rating specialists reported that many disability cases now require rating by analogy, and that the number of these cases is increasing. The GAO also identified 15 medical conditions not listed in the Rating Schedule and asked rating specialists to list the analogous codes they could use to rate the 15 conditions. Rating specialists reported that at least 10 different diagnostic codes could be used for each of the medical conditions.

The GAO study demonstrated that veterans were given different ratings dependent on the subjective judgment of the rating specialists. For example, 60% of the respondents selected a diagnostic code for Crohn's disease with degrees of severity ranging from 10 to 100%.

This study concluded that the vagueness and generality of the Rating Schedule contributed to the lack of uniformity between rating boards in rating disabilities.

In one study reviewed by the GAO, VA raters were presented with disability cases representing 23 separate impairments for which veterans had already been awarded VA disability compensation benefits. All relevant medical information necessary to decide on a rating was taken from the case files. Copies were then sent to rating boards at 56 of the 58 VA regional offices participating in the assessment. At each location, one or more rating boards (or a combination of board members) assigned disability ratings using the medical information supplied for the 23 impairments, the study showed that:

- 11 were assigned two different ratings;
- 6 were assigned three different ratings;
- 4 were assigned four different ratings; and
- 2 were assigned five different ratings.

The study authors identified two areas where the judgment of the rating specialists may result in ratings that are particularly inconsistent.

First of all, the Rating Schedule includes many diagnostic codes with minimal medical criteria (such as "severe" or "moderate") to distinguish between degrees of severity. In these situations, the rating specialist must subjectively decide which degree of severity is supported by medical findings.

Secondly, a medical examination may identify a medical condition that is not listed in the Schedule. The rating specialist must then rate by analogy, as mentioned earlier, and select a diagnostic code that has symptoms similar to the identified medical condition.

In 2007, the VA invited the Institute of Medicine (IOM) to review its rating system and recommend an update of the Schedule. The committee, chaired by the then President of the American Medical Association, reviewed the rating table and stated:

> "This IOM Committee on Medical Evaluation of Veterans for Disability Compensation notes in its report that our nation's veterans' benefits program has not kept a similar pace of progress in understanding disability…The original concern for the sacrifices made by those who serve our nation's colors had its genesis in the Revolutionary War, when loss of limbs, eyes, or other body parts sharply reduced a person's ability to support himself. This emphasis on anatomical loss persisted through the 19th century, was codified in the Rating Schedule

developed to implement the War Risk Insurance Act of 1917, and retained with modifications in subsequent Rating Schedules, including the current one when it was developed in 1945. The architecture put in place at that time has been updated from time to time in a piecemeal manner, and some sections are largely the same as in 1945. There has been resistance to change what was known and comfortable, which is understandable, but this should not stand in the way of our ability to evaluate and compensate for disability based on up- to-date medical knowledge of impairment and function."

The Rating Schedule of 1945 remains largely unchanged since its conception. It mainly focused on young soldiers returning from World War II and emphasized loss of limbs and restrictions of movement rather than disability as determined by the American Medical Association dictionary of impairment or the criteria used by the Social Security Administration.

As the IOM committee noted, the Rating Schedule ignores the importance of imaging technology, which was not available in 1945, and ignores significant medical advances since 1945. For example, the Rating Schedule defines incapacitating episodes for back pain as periods of acute symptoms that requires a doctor's prescription for bed-rest. The treatment of back pain by bed-rest has been abandoned. The American College of Physicians and the American Pain Society provided the following guidelines for the treatment of back pain (excerpts are from Diagnosis and Treatment of Low

Back Pain: A Joint Clinical Practice Guideline from the American College of Physicians and the American Pain Society Ann Intern Med. 2007;147:478-491):

> "General advice on self-management for nonspecific low back pain should include recommendations to remain active, which is more effective than resting in bed for patients with acute or subacute low back pain (65, 66). If patients require periods of bed rest to relieve severe symptoms, they should be encouraged to return to normal activities as soon as possible."

Instead of bedrest, the panel recommended:

> "Recommendation 7: For patients who do not improve with self-care options, clinicians should consider the addition of nonpharmacologic therapy with proven benefits for acute low back pain, spinal manipulation; for chronic or subacute low back pain, intensive interdisciplinary rehabilitation, exercise therapy, acupuncture, massage therapy, spinal manipulation, yoga, cognitive-behavioral therapy, or progressive relaxation (weak recommendation, moderate-quality evidence)."

It appears that even the Veterans' Administration has accepted these recommendations, as they have been included in in a VA training letter to its staff.

Finally, unlike the young soldiers of World War II, current veterans have aged; many are veterans of the

Vietnam War and suffer from degenerative diseases secondary to their injuries several decades earlier. They suffer from numerous internal medicine diseases including sleep apnea, heart, liver and lung disease, often not directly related to the service but secondary to other service-connected injuries. The Rating Schedule of 1945 can hardly do justice in evaluating their claims.

CHAPTER 2 – INDEPENDENT MEDICAL OPINION (IMO) AND NEXUS LETTERS FOR DISABLED VETERANS

What is a Nexus?

There are three steps involved in a claim for service connection according to *Caluza v. Brown*, 7 Vet. App. 498. First, the veteran must present satisfactory lay or other evidence of service incurrence or aggravation of such injury or disease [38 U.S.C.S. 1154(b)]. Second, the VA must determine whether that evidence is consistent with the circumstances, conditions, or hardships of such service. The third and final requirement is demonstrating that there is a nexus (a link or a connection) between the current disability (requirement #1) and the precipitating disease, injury, or event that occurred during the period of military service (requirement #2).

What is an Independent Medical Opinion (IMO)?

To meet the nexus requirement, a veteran must have an evaluation by a physician that will establish that the veteran is indeed disabled and that his disability is as likely as not caused by his military service.

There are two methods used to establish such a nexus. One is an Independent Medical Examination (IME) and the other is an Independent Medical Opinion (IMO). An IME involves an actual examination of the veteran at a doctor's office. An IMO does not require a physical examination, but does require that an experienced physician carefully review the entire medical record and the C&P examinations, and then perform independent and thorough medical research relevant to the issues of the veteran's case.

Why Do Veterans Need an IMO/ Nexus Letter?

The Institute of Medicine (IOM) was asked by the Veterans' Disability Benefits Commission to study and recommend improvements in the medical evaluation and rating of veterans for the benefits provided by the Department of Veterans Affairs (VA) to compensate for illnesses or injuries incurred in or aggravated by military service.

The IOM noted inadequacies in the qualifications of the raters employed by the VA:

> "Few raters have medical backgrounds. They are required to review and assess medical evidence provided by treating physicians and VHA examining physicians and determine percentage of disability, but VBA does not have medical consultants or advisers to support the raters. Medical advisers would also improve the process of deciding what medical examinations and tests are needed to sufficiently prepare a case for rating."

The IOM reported that 24% (95,000 of 405,000) of the Compensation and Pension (C&P) examinations were incomplete in FY 1993, a percentage that had not improved much in FY 1996, when 22% were incomplete (VA, 1997b).

The IOM also found that of the spine exams requested during the second quarter of fiscal year 2005, 32% of the exam requests had at least one error, such as not identifying the pertinent condition or not requesting the appropriate exam.

Requirements for an Adequate Medical Opinion - Why is a Veteran's Primary Physician's Opinion Often Insufficient?

James D. Ridgway was a Senior Law Clerk for a member of the United States Court of Appeals for Veterans Claims. He wrote an excellent article on this subject entitled "Lessons the Veterans Benefits System Must Learn on Gathering Expert Witness Evidence". The article is based on his thorough knowledge of the veteran disability system as well in depth research of the relevant legal case law and statutes. The following are excerpts from his work:

> "At the most basic level, an adequate medical opinion is one that allows the VA adjudicator's "evaluation of the claimed disability [to] be a fully informed one." The standard is only understood by looking at how the evidence will be evaluated. A defining characteristic of the VA adjudication system is that the initial decision-makers at the fifty-seven regional offices ("ROs") are neither medical professionals nor attorneys. Because VA adjudicators are not medical

professionals, an adequate opinion is one that can be weighed and evaluated by a layperson...

Although a veteran enjoys the benefit of the doubt, the adjudicator may not be willing to grant benefits based upon speculation that a current condition is related to service. In practice, this means that a letter from the veteran's doctor stating merely that he or she believes that the veteran's current condition is related to some in-service injury or disease will not be sufficient to grant benefits. An adjudicator cannot simply rely on the assertion of a veteran's treating physician.

Rather, the medical opinion must provide sufficient detail to make clear its factual basis and the theory of causation, and thereby convince the adjudicator that there is a basis for granting the claim. An adequate medical opinion must meet numerous criteria. First, the opinion should state its factual premise in detail, including the precise nature of the in-service disease or injury and whether there have been any intervening post-service injuries or diseases. This statement of facts should indicate its sources, including to what extent the facts are taken from available medical records, versus history supplied by the veteran. The degree to which an opinion discusses and accounts for the veteran's documented medical history is a relevant factor. VA may reject a medical opinion as having no value because of an inaccurate factual premise, and an incomplete factual premise diminishes the weight that the opinion might otherwise be assigned.

Second, the opinion should state the diagnosis of the veteran's current condition. The opinion should list each symptom attributable to the veteran's current condition and when the condition first manifested. The physician should also document any objective test results supporting the existence, severity, or duration of any symptom. If applicable, the opinion should note specifically whether the veteran's symptoms have been continuous since service. If the condition is chronic, the opinion should discuss whether the available evidence is sufficient to determine that the condition first manifested as chronic during service. If appropriate, it should also address prior conflicting diagnoses and the possibility that some symptoms may be attributable to a different condition.

Third, the medical opinion should state why the physician believes that the veteran's condition relates to service. The physician must state this opinion in terms that make clear that the expert believes that it is at least as likely as not that a relationship exists. If the theory of causation is not generally accepted in the medical community, then it may be necessary for the doctor to note any research that was conducted and what authorities support the stated theory of causation. A medical opinion should address prior negative opinions, and the rationale for rejecting a contrary opinion is an important factor when a lay adjudicator is weighing the evidence.

Additionally, the Secretary's duty to assist requires that he obtain an opinion that discusses every theory of causation raised by the record. Therefore, one of the most frequent reasons that VA rejects an opinion is that the opinion addresses only direct service connection without analyzing whether there was continuity of symptomatology, secondary service connection, or another alternative theory.

It may seem at first blush that the requirements are somewhat onerous, but it is important to remember that they are neutral. Although they may make it difficult for a private physician to provide an opinion in support of a claim, these requirements also make it difficult for VA to deny a claim based upon a less than thorough opinion. Ultimately, the purpose of the requirements is to make sure the decision is reliable regardless of outcome. However, it is easy to see why it may be difficult for a private physician to provide a medical opinion that is adequate to support an award of benefits. Unless a doctor has experience testifying as an expert, he or she may not understand how much detail is necessary to provide a medical opinion that is adequate and persuasive to a lay VA adjudicator. What is more difficult to understand is how the VA has reached the 21st century without developing procedures for assisting private physicians to render adequate opinions for the veterans that they treat."

The Importance of Published Medical Reports (Treatises) in an IMO

Proving a nexus between a veteran's disability and his military service requires both factual and scientific evidence. In most cases, especially for the veterans who served in Vietnam, service records are difficult to obtain; most records have been either damaged or lost. Without these records, it is difficult to prove that a current disability was caused by injuries that occurred 40 or 50 years ago.

Most veterans, however, have already established service connection for some disabilities and the question is usually whether their current disabling condition is related to the service-connected disabilities. The determination of secondary disability is no longer factual, but rather strictly a scientific question. A veteran only needs to show that the scientific community supports his claim that condition x is related to his service-connected disabilities. To deny a veteran's claim, the VA must have an equally qualified scientist state that there is no scientific connection between the claimed condition and the service-connected conditions. Even then, the VA must accept the IMO based on the benefit of the doubt doctrine.

The Veteran's Court has held that a medical article or treatise "can provide important support when combined with an opinion of a medical professional" if the medical article or treatise evidence discusses generic relationships with a degree of certainty such that, under the facts of a specific case, there is at least "plausible causality" based upon objective facts rather than on an unsubstantiated lay medical opinion. *Mattern v. West*, 12 Vet. App. 222, 228 (1999); see also *Sacks v. West*, 11 Vet. App. 314 (1998) and *Wallin v. West*, 11 Vet. App. 509 (1998)

A submission of a scientific report, even by a layperson, requires the Board to address the report, or medical treatise.

In a decision rendered by Judge Bartley in *Bowers v. Shinseki* No. 11-3022, the judge was critical of the BVA's failure to address medical treatises provided by the veteran. The BVA held that such reports were merely layperson's opinion. Judge Bartley held, "As a layperson, the Veteran is not competent generally to render a probative opinion on a medical matter. Mr. Bowers, however, was not offering his own subjective opinion as to the growth rate of gallstones; he was repeating the data reported in professional medical treatises he submitted. Certainly, a layperson is competent to report information provided by a medical professional. Cf. *Jandreau v. Nicholson*, 492 F.3d 1372, 1377 (Fed. Cir.2007) (ruling that a veteran is competent to repeat a medical diagnosis and report observable symptoms).

In labeling the veteran's report of the growth rate of gallstones as incompetent lay opinion, the Board avoided addressing the substance of the medical treatise evidence Mr. Bowers submitted, just as the Board failed to address those treatises directly. Thus, the Board's failure to address the medical treatise evidence that was favorable to Mr. Bowers was not harmless."

BVA Decision Held that Obstructive Sleep Apnea (OSA) is Secondary to Posttraumatic Stress Disorder (PTSD) Based on this Author's IMO

DOCKET No. 11-01 922   Date: 03/28/2016

"A June 2014 letter from Dr. D. Anaise included an opinion that the Veteran's sleep apnea was more likely than not secondary to his service-connected PTSD. The letter cited medical literature as evidence in support of the opinion, and included such medical literature in support of the Veteran's claim. Such evidence was also in support of a causal relationship between sleep apnea and PTSD.

After a review of the evidence of record, resolving all reasonable doubt in the veteran's favor, the Board finds that the preponderance of the evidence supports that the Veteran's obstructive sleep apnea is secondary to his service-connected PTSD...

The Board notes that the September 2012 VA opinion against the Veteran's claim cited the lack of medical literature in support of a causal relationship between PTSD and sleep apnea as a basis for concluding the Veteran's sleep apnea was less likely as not caused by or a result of his PTSD. In contrast, the June 2014 letter from Dr. D. Anaise indicated there was a significant volume of medical literature to support the Veteran's claim, and cited to such evidence in support of his opinion that the Veteran's obstructive sleep apnea was more likely than not secondary to his service-connected PTSD. The Board finds the June 2014 letter and opinion from Dr. D. Anaise to be more probative and persuasive in this case as it was based on a review of the Veteran's treatment records, cited supporting medical literature, and was provided by a medical expert competent to provide an opinion as to the etiology of the Veteran's sleep apnea. Hence, entitlement to service connection for obstructive sleep apnea as secondary to service-connected PTSD is warranted."

BVA Decision Held that OSA is Secondary to Asthma Based on this Author's IMO

DOCKET No. 11-08 722   Date: 02/08/2016

"The Veteran's attorney, who is a physician, provided a statement that related the Veteran's sleep apnea to his asthma. This statement cited medical literature in support of this conclusion and provided a description of the process by which asthma can result in sleep apnea.

The Board finds that the medical evidence for and against the claim is at least in relative equipoise. Resolving reasonable doubt in favor of the Veteran, there is a basis of entitlement to service connection on a secondary basis under 38 C.F.R.§ 3.310. See 38 U.S.C.A.§5107(b); 38 C.F.R. §3.102."

CHAPTER 3 - TOTAL DISABILITY BASED ON INDIVIDUAL UNEMPLOYABILITY (TDIU)

It is VA policy that all veterans who are unable to secure and follow a substantially gainful occupation due to service-connected disabilities shall be rated totally disabled. 38 C.F.R. § 4.16(b). The VA defines unemployability as follows [40 FR 42536, Sept. 15, 1975, as amended at 43 FR 45349, Oct. 2, 1978]:

> "A veteran may be considered as unemployable upon termination of employment which was provided because disability, or in which special consideration was given on account of the same, when it is satisfactorily shown that he or she is unable to secure further employment… However, consideration is to be given to the circumstances of employment in individual claims, and, if the employment was only occasional, intermittent, try out or unsuccessful, or eventually terminated on account of the disability, present unemployability may be attributed to the static disability."

TDIU Requires that a Veteran Be Unable to Secure Substantially Gainful Occupation

The VA has defined substantially gainful occupation in its Adjudication Procedures Manual (Manual M21-1MR, Part VI, subpart ii, 2F.24.d) as that which is ordinarily followed by the nondisabled to earn their livelihood with earnings common to the particular occupation in the community where the veteran resides. Marginal employment is not considered substantially gainful employment. Marginal employment is defined as earned annual income that does not exceed the poverty threshold for one person as established by the U.S. Department of Commerce, Bureau of the Census. Under the current poverty threshold established by the Bureau of the Census, marginal income for the year 2010 is $11,334.00.

In *Faust v. West*, (13 Vet. App. 342, 356 (2000), the Court adopted a definition of a substantially gainful occupation. The Court concluded that a "substantially gainful occupation is [an occupation] that provides [the veteran with an] annual income that exceeds the poverty threshold for one person, irrespective of the number of hours or days that the veteran actually works."

In *Roberson v. Principi*, (251 F.3d 1378, 1385 (Fed. Cir. 2001), the Federal Circuit further defined that the term "substantially gainful activity" (SGA) is flexible. Although the term SGA may not set a clear numerical standard for determining TDIU, it does indicate an amount less than 100%. A veteran, because of service-connected disability, must be incapable of performing the physical and mental acts required by employment; the question is not whether he can find employment. *Van Hoose,* 4 Vet. App. at 363. "[T]he BVA may not reject [a veteran's] claim without producing evidence, *as distinguished from mere conjecture*, that the veteran can perform work that would produce sufficient income to be other than marginal." *Bowling v. Principi*, 15 Vet.App. 1, 9 (2001) (emphasis in text) quoting *Beaty v. Brown*, 6 Vet.App. 532, 539 (1994) citing *see also James v. Brown*, 7 Vet.App. 495, 497 (1995) ("The

Board 'was not convinced that there were not some jobs he could do' but no evidence supported that conclusion")

The VA will grant a total rating for compensation purposes based on unemployability when the evidence shows that the veteran is precluded, by reason of his service-connected disabilities, from obtaining and maintaining any form of gainful employment consistent with education and occupational experience.

Under the applicable regulations, benefits based on individual unemployability are granted only when it is established that the service-connected disabilities are so severe, standing alone, as to prevent the retaining of gainful employment. Under 38 C.F.R. § 4.16, if there is only one such disability, it must be rated at least 60% disabling to qualify for benefits based on individual unemployability. If there are two or more such disabilities, there shall be at least one disability ratable at 40% or more and sufficient additional disability to bring the combined rating to 70% or more. 38 C.F.R. § 4.16(a).

In a pertinent precedent opinion, the VA General Counsel concluded that the controlling VA regulations generally provide that veterans who, in light of their individual circumstances, but without regard to age, are unable to secure and follow a substantially gainful occupation as the result of service-connected disability shall be rated totally disabled, without regard to whether an average person would be rendered unemployable by the circumstances. Thus, the criteria include a subjective standard. It was also determined that "unemployability" is synonymous with inability to secure and follow a substantially gainful occupation. VAOPGCPREC 75-91 (O.G.C. Prec. 75-91); 57 Fed. Reg. 2,317 (1992).

Individual Unemployability - Consideration of Educational and Occupational History

When evaluating a veteran's employability, consideration may be given to his/her level of education, special training, and previous work experience, but not to age or impairment caused by non-service-connected disabilities. 38 C.F.R. §§ 3.341, 4.19

Once a Veteran is found to have 60% service-connected disability (or 40%/70%) in step one of the analysis, the VA analyzes the veteran's educational and occupational history to determine whether his service-connected disabilities preclude him from securing or following substantially gainful employment (activity) (SGA).

In *Beaty v. Brown*, 6 Vet. App. 532, 537 (1994), the Court held that to determine whether service-connected disability precludes SGA, a general medical examination is to be scheduled in which the examiner is requested to provide an opinion as to whether or not it is at least as likely as not that the veteran's service-connected disability or combined disabilities render him or her unable to secure and maintain SGA, to include describing the disabilities' functional impairment and how that impairment impacts on physical and sedentary employment. See also VA Training Letter 10-07 (Sept. 14, 2010).

The Court has stated:

> "[w]here the veteran submits a claim for a TDIU rating ... the BVA may not reject that claim without producing evidence, as distinguished from mere conjecture, that the veteran can perform work that would produce sufficient income to be other than marginal."

The simple fact that a veteran may be young, or may be highly educated, or may have been recently employed, or may have had a long work career are not decisive, and standing alone are insufficient justifications to deny a TDIU claim; *Gleicher v. Derwinski*, 2 Vet. App. 26 (1992).

What is the Effective Date for TDIU?

The General Counsel provided a binding opinion in VAOPGCPREC 12-2001 regarding *Roberson v. Principi*, No. 00-7009, 2001 U.S. App. LEXIS 11008 (Fed. Cir. May 29, 2001), holding the following:

1. Once a veteran: (1) submits evidence of a medical disability; (2) makes a claim for the highest rating possible; and (3) submits evidence of unemployability, the requirement in 38 C.F.R. 3.155(a) that an informal claim "identify the benefit sought" has been satisfied and the VA must consider whether the veteran

is entitled to total disability based upon individual unemployability (TDIU).

2. A veteran is not required to submit proof that he or she is 100% unemployable in order to establish an inability to maintain a substantially gainful occupation, as required for a TDIU award pursuant to 38 C.F.R. 3.340(a).

The VA often demands that a veteran first file for TDIU and assign the onset date as the date the veteran filed for TDIU or filed VA Form 21-8940. This is an error. When a veteran files an original claim for evaluation of a disability or a claim for an increase in the evaluation of a disability that has already been rated by the VA, the claimant is generally presumed to be seeking the highest benefit allowable. (See *AB v. Brown*, 6 Vet. App. 35, 38 (1983); see also *Roberson v. Principi*, 251 F.3d 1378, 1383 (Fed. Cir. 2001); *Rice v. Shinseki*, 22 Vet. App. 447 (2009); *Norris v. West*, 12 Vet. App. 413, 421 (1999). If either claim includes facts that indicate that the veteran is unemployable, the VA is obligated to consider and adjudicate a TDIU claim.

In *Servello v. Derwinski*, 3 Vet. App. 196 (1992), the Court held that the existence of an inferred claim for TDIU might have entitled the veteran to an earlier effective date because under 38 U.S.C.S. 5110(b)(2), the effective date of an award of increased compensation shall be the earliest date as of which it is ascertainable that an increase in disability occurred if the application is received within one year from such date. The court reasoned that because under 38 C.F.R. 3.155(a), the VA was required to, but did not, forward to the veteran a TDIU application form, the one-year filing period for such application did not begin to run. Thus, as a matter of law, the inferred claim submitted prior to the date of a formal TDIU application must be accepted as the date of claim for effective date purposes.

In *Collier v. Derwinski*, 2 Vet. App. 247, 251 (1992), the Court held the VA was obliged to consider the issue of entitlement to TDIU benefits despite the veteran not having filed the specific TDIU application form because he has continually stated that he is unable to work due to his schizophrenia. *Roberson*, 251 F.3d at 1384; *Norris*, 12 Vet. App. at 421.

In *Rice v. Shinseki*, 22 Vet. App. 447 (2009) the CAVC concluded:

> "The Court holds that a request for TDIU is best understood as part of an initial claim for VA disability compensation based on the individual effect of the veteran's underlying disability or disabilities or as a particular type of claim for increased compensation. This is not to say that a claimant cannot submit a request for TDIU at any time, whether on a VA Form 21-8940 or in any other manner. Submission of a request for TDIU does not change the essential character of an assertion of entitlement to TDIU as a part of either an initial claim or a claim for increase."

In *Rice v. Shinseki*, 22 Vet. App. 447 (2009), the Court made it clear that the Veterans' Administration has a duty to investigate the eligibility of a veteran for TDIU when the veteran requests a higher rating which will entitle him/her to schedular unemployability and the records indicate evidence of unemployability. The Court stated:

> "It is clear from our jurisprudence that an initial claim for benefits for a particular disability might also include an assertion of entitlement to TDIU based on that disability (**either overtly stated or implied by a fair reading of the claim or of the evidence of record**) (emphasis added)…The Federal Circuit's recent decision in *Comer v. Peake* contains language consistent with this analysis: "A claim to TDIU benefits is not a free-standing claim that must be pled with specificity; it is implicitly raised whenever a pro se veteran, who presents cogent evidence of unemployability, seeks to obtain a higher disability rating." 552 F.3d 1362, 1367 (Fed. Cir. 2009). This statement of the law is consistent with and reiterated the Federal Circuit's earlier decision in *Roberson v. Prinicpi*, involving the assignment of an initial disability rating, which reversed this Court's holding that Mr. Roberson failed to make "a claim for TDIU" and held that consideration of TDIU is required once "a veteran submits evidence of a medical disability and makes a claim for the highest rating possible, and additionally submits evidence of unemployability." 251 F.3d 1378, 1384 (Fed. Cir.

2001); see also Bernklau v. Principi, 291 F.3d 795, 799 (Fed. Cir. 2002) (discussing a request for TDIU in the context of a claim for increased compensation for an already service- connected disability). Further, this Court has already stated this principal clearly: "A TDIU rating is not a basis for an award of service connection. Rather, it is merely an alternate way to obtain a total disability rating without being rated 100% disabled under the Rating Schedule." Norris v. West, 12 Vet.App. 413, 420-21(1999). Considering the facts of Comer, Robertson, Bernklau, and Norris, we hold that a request for TDIU, whether expressly raised by a veteran or reasonably raised by the record, is not a separate claim for benefits, but rather involves an attempt to obtain an appropriate rating for a disability or disabilities, either as part of the initial adjudication of a claim or as part of a claim for increased compensation, where the disability upon which entitlement to TDIU is based has already been found to be service-connected."

Is VA Form 21-8940 "Veteran's Application for Increased Compensation Based on Unemployability" Mandatory in a TDIU claim?

VA rating decisions almost always state that the veteran is not entitled to unemployability because he did not provide *VA Form 21-8940*. This is contrary to the VA's established policy. As M21-1MR Section F clearly shows, (Date September 15, 2011):

> "*Note*: Although a *VA Form 21-8940* can be an important development tool, it is not required to render a decision in an IU claim"

While VA Form 21-8940 is not mandatory, and clearly should not be the basis for denial of a veteran's right to benefits, it is recommended that veterans submit the form with their appeal.

What is the Effect of a Favorable Social Security Disability Decision on a Veteran's Disability Claim?

If the Social Security Administration (SSA) finds that a veteran is unable to secure any job in the national economy, is that decision binding on the VA?

A favorable rating decision by the VA is entitled to evidentiary weight in a Social Security hearing. In *Thomas E. McCartey v. Massanari*, 298 F.3d 1072 9th Circ 2002, the Court agreed that a VA disability rating is entitled to evidentiary weight in a Social Security hearing. See *Chambliss v. Massanari*, 269 F.3d 520, 522 (5th Cir.2001) (per curiam) (VA disability rating is generally entitled to "great weight" and "must be considered by the ALJ"):

> "We so conclude because of the marked similarity between these two federal disability programs. Both programs serve the same governmental purpose — providing benefits to those unable to work because of a serious disability. Both programs evaluate a claimant's

ability to perform full-time work in the national economy on a sustained and continuing basis; both focus on analyzing a claimant's functional limitations; and both require claimants to present extensive medical documentation in support of their claims. Compare 38 C.F.R. § 4.1 et seq. (VA ratings) with 20 C.F.R. § 404.1 et seq (Social Security Disability). Both programs have a detailed regulatory scheme that promotes consistency in adjudication of claims. Both are administered by the federal government, and they share a common incentive to weed out meritless claims."

SSA decisions regarding a veteran's unemployability are "pertinent," but not controlling, in a VA disability claim. *Murincsak v. Derwinski*, 2 Vet. App. 363 (1992). Since the SSA and the VA define unemployability somewhat differently, the SSA's decision will not always mirror the VA's.

The relevant factor is whether the SSA's decision was based on service-connected disabilities. Since it is not always clear whether the SSA's decision is based on service-connected or non-service-connected disabilities, there are sometimes cases where the VA will not give the SSA's determination as much weight. VA rules prevent the VA from giving weight to non-service-connected disabilities or age, while both factors often play prominent roles in the SSA's decision.

The VA cannot simply ignore a favorable decision by the SSA. It must determine whether the SSA made its decision based on the veteran's service-connected disability or non–service-connected disability. In *Quartuccio v. Principi*, 16 Vet. App. 183, 187-88 (2002), the Court held in a psychiatric disability benefits case where SSA benefits had been granted for a psychiatric disability, a remand to obtain Social Security records were required where the "possibility that the SSA records could contain relevant evidence ... cannot be foreclosed absent a review of those records."

CHAPTER 4 – SLEEP APNEA

Service-connected Conditions That Cause Obstructive Sleep Apnea (OSA)

The number of veterans and military retirees receiving disability compensation from the VA for sleep apnea has skyrocketed in recent years.

In 2012, the number of veterans and retirees receiving compensation for sleep apnea was 114,103, almost double the number the VA reported in 2009 (57,679). The number of veterans added to the rolls from 2001 to 2012 increased 25-fold. 983 veterans obtained disability compensation for sleep apnea in 2001. In 2012, 24,791 veterans were added to the rolls to treat the condition, according to a report by Tom Philpott in the military publication Stars and Stripes.

A review of BVA decisions show that 3 out of every 4 veterans **will be denied** service connection for their sleep apnea claim by the BVA.

Most claims for sleep apnea are denied based on two arguments. The first is that the veteran was not diagnosed as suffering from sleep apnea during service. The second is that sleep apnea is caused by obesity, and since members of the armed forces are uniformly fit, a veteran could not possibly have suffered from sleep apnea during their military service, but rather gained weight, and thus, became susceptible to sleep apnea in civilian life.

To the first argument, I respond that sleep apnea was not even recognized as a medical entity prior to 1994. Between 1992-1993, the congressionally appointed National Commission on Sleep Disorders Research, chaired by Dr. William C. Dement, discovered that there is a startling lack of information about sleep disorders among general practitioners. This lack of information has resulted in numerous misdiagnoses and mistreatments of patients, estimated in the millions. In many of these cases, a little knowledge and the right treatment might have worked wonders. Because of the Commission's work, legislation to create a National Center for Sleep Disorders Research was passed into law in January 1993.

As for the second argument, it is true that obesity is often associated with sleep apnea, however, that does not change the fact that there are numerous medical conditions that do cause sleep apnea.

It is my firm belief that it is futile to attempt to prove that sleep apnea is based directly on military service. Instead, I advise veterans to show that sleep apnea is secondary to other service-connected disabilities; OSA secondary to:

- Sinusitis, Rhinitis, Deviated Septum (p. 56)
- PTSD (p. 59)
- Chronic Pain Syndrome (p. 66)

- Narcotics (p. 69)
- Tinnitus (p. 71)
- Chronic Obstructive Pulmonary Disease (COPD)/Asthma (p. 74)
- Gastroesophageal Reflux Disease (GERD) (p. 78)
- Diabetes Mellitus (p. 82)
- Stroke and Ischemic Heart Disease (p. 84)
- Cervical Spine Abnormalities (p. 85)
- Fibromyalgia (p. 89)
- Upper Airway Resistance Syndrome (UARS) (p. 90)
- Antidepressants (p. 92)
- Interstitial Lung Disease (p. 95)
- Cardiovascular Disease (CVD) (p. 97)
- Headaches/Migraines (p. 100)

When a medical expert provides such analysis, and encloses treatises that show uniform support by the scientific community as to the existence of such a relationship, the BVA, as a matter of law, is required to accept such analysis unless it can produce a more forceful scientific argument to defeat this opinion.

What is Obstructive Sleep Apnea?

Obstructive sleep apnea (OSA) is a sleep disorder that involves cessation or significant decrease in airflow in the presence of breathing effort. It is the most common type of sleep-disordered breathing and is characterized by recurrent episodes of upper airway collapse during sleep. These episodes are associated with recurrent oxyhemoglobin desaturations and arousals from sleep. Generally, symptoms of OSA begin insidiously and are often present for years before the patient is referred for evaluation.

Nocturnal symptoms may include the following: snoring, usually loud, habitual, and bothersome to others; witnessed apneas, which often interrupt the snoring and end with a snort; insomnia; restless sleep, with patients often experiencing frequent arousals and tossing or turning during the night.

Daytime symptoms may include the following: non-restorative sleep (i.e. "waking up as tired as when they went to bed"); morning headache; dry or sore throat; excessive daytime sleepiness that usually begins during quiet activities (e.g. reading, watching television).

As the severity worsens, patients begin to feel sleepy during activities that generally require alertness (e.g., school, work, driving). Patients begin to experience: daytime fatigue/tiredness; cognitive deficits; memory and intellectual impairment (short-term memory, concentration); decreased vigilance; morning confusion; personality and mood changes, including depression and anxiety; sexual dysfunction, including impotence and decreased libido; gastroesophageal reflux and hypertension.

A sleep-related breathing disorder (SRBD) continuum has been described and is supported by research. OSA can be thought of as occupying a range of this continuum. The SRBD continuum suggests that snoring is the initial presenting symptom and it increases in severity over time. It also increases in association with medical disorders that may serve to exacerbate the disorder, such as obesity. Snoring has a constellation of pathophysiological effects. As the disease progresses, SRBD patients begin to develop increased UA (Upper Airway) resistance that results in a new hallmark symptom: sleepiness. Sleepiness is caused by increased arousals from sleep.

Rating for Sleep Apnea

6847 Sleep Apnea Syndromes (Obstructive, Central, Mixed)	% Disabled
Chronic respiratory failure with carbon dioxide retention or cor pulmonale; or requires tracheostomy	100
Requires use of breathing assistance device such as continuous airway pressure (CPAP) machine	50
Persistent day-time hypersomnolence	30
Asymptomatic but with documented sleep disorder breathing	0

OSA (ICD-9-CM 327.23) is the most common form of sleep apnea and is caused by an airway blockage that occurs when the soft tissue in the back of the throat narrows or closes during sleep. The brain then senses the inability to breathe and briefly arouses the person to begin breathing again.

Central sleep apnea (ICD –9-CM 327.27) occurs when the brain doesn't send proper signals to the muscles that control breathing, and the person may awaken with shortness of breath.

Complex or mixed sleep apnea is a combination of both obstructive and central sleep apnea.

For rating purposes, the rating table does not distinguish between obstructive, central and mixed sleep apnea. Pure obstructive sleep apnea involves abnormalities of the upper airway such as enlarged tonsils, large tongue or blocked nasal passages. Yet, in all these cases there is no mechanical blockage to the airway during wakefulness and obstruction occurs only during sleep. The reason for sleep apnea in these cases is that the brain does not send proper signals to the muscles that control breathing.

Thus, all sleep apnea cases are in fact mixed sleep apnea. Obstructive sleep apnea has become the term of art for all sleep apnea. I have yet to encounter a single case where the diagnosis of sleep apnea did not carry the diagnosis of obstructive sleep apnea, rather than central or mixed.

Development of Sleep Apnea During Military Service

To prove that sleep apnea developed during military service, a veteran typically submits statements to the VA attesting to the fact that he/she snored and experienced daytime fatigue while in service. Veterans also provide corroborative statements from former military service roommates.

Dr. Ralph Downey III, PhD, in his article, *Obstructive Sleep Apnea,* reports:

> "Obstructive sleep apnea (OSA) — also referred to as obstructive sleep apnea-hypopnea — is a sleep disorder that involves cessation or significant decrease in airflow in the presence of breathing effort. It is the most common type of sleep-disordered breathing and is characterized by recurrent episodes of upper airway collapse during sleep. These episodes are associated with recurrent oxyhemoglobin desaturations and arousals from sleep…"
>
> Generally, symptoms of OSA begin insidiously and are often present for years before the patient is referred for evaluation.
>
> Nocturnal symptoms may include the following:
>
> - Snoring, usually loud, habitual, and bothersome to others
> - Witnessed apneas, which often interrupt the snoring and end with a snort…

- Insomnia; restless sleep, with patients often experiencing frequent tossing or turning during the night

Daytime symptoms may include the following:

- Nonrestorative sleep (i.e., "waking up as tired as when they went to bed")
- Excessive daytime sleepiness that usually begins during quiet activities (egg, reading, watching television); as the severity worsens, patients begin to feel sleepy during activities that generally require alertness (e.g., school, work, driving)
- Daytime fatigue/tiredness

A sleep-related breathing disorder (SRBD) continuum has been described and is supported by research. OSA can be thought of as occupying a range of this continuum.

The SRBD continuum suggests that snoring is the initial presenting symptom, and it increases in severity over time and it increases in association with medical disorders that may serve to exacerbate the disorder, such as obesity. Snoring has a constellation of pathophysiological effects.

As the disease progresses, SRBD patients begin to develop increased UA (upper airway) resistance that results in a new hallmark symptom: sleepiness. Sleepiness is caused by increased arousals from sleep. This syndrome has been described as the UA resistance syndrome (UARS). UARS patients are not hypoxic, and hypoxia does not explain why they are sleepy, nor can sleep stage percentages or other polysomnography (PSG) variables. The SRBD continuum predicts that over time, a UARS patient develops OSA, if untreated..."

Snoring is the initial presenting symptom on the sleep-related breathing disorder (SRBD) continuum. As the disease progresses, SRBD patients begin to show sleepiness, due to increased upper airway resistance. If untreated, the patient eventually develops Obstructive Sleep Apnea (OSA) with symptoms of snoring, sleepiness, spouse apnea report, and hypoxia.

Persuaded by this author's IMO, the BVA has acknowledged the connection between snoring to the development of sleep apnea in its decision of February 28, 2016 (Docket No. 11-08 722).

Sleep Apnea Secondary to Service-Connected Sinusitis, Rhinitis or Deviated Septum

Upper respiratory conditions (sinusitis) result in distortion of the upper airway, which contributes to the development of sleep apnea.

Conceptually, the upper airway is a compliant tube and, therefore, is subject to collapse. OSA is caused by soft tissue collapse in the pharynx. Transmural pressure is the difference between intraluminal pressure and the surrounding tissue pressure. If transmural pressure decreases, the cross-sectional area of the pharynx decreases. If this pressure passes a critical point, pharyngeal closing pressure is reached. Exceeding pharyngeal critical pressure (Pcrit) causes a juggernaut of tissues collapsing inward. The airway is then obstructed. Until forces change transmural pressure to a net tissue force that is less than Pcrit, the airway remains obstructed.

OSA duration is equal to the time that Pcrit is exceeded. The Bernoulli effect plays an important dynamic role in OSA pathophysiology. In accordance with this effect, airflow velocity increases at the site of stricture in the airway. As airway velocity increases, pressure on the lateral wall decreases. If the transmural closing pressure is reached, the airway collapses.

The Bernoulli effect is exaggerated in areas where the airway is most compliant. Loads on the pharyngeal walls increase adherence and, hence, increase the likelihood of collapse. This effect helps to partially explain why obese patients, and particularly those with fat deposition in the neck, are most likely to have OSA. Given this information, it is abundantly clear that even a small reduction in a diameter of the upper airway will cause a collapse of the upper airway during sleep.

Fitzpatrick et al. studied the effect of nasal breathing on sleep apnea in the article *Effect of nasal or oral breathing route on upper airway resistance during sleep*. The author reports that healthy subjects with normal nasal resistance breathe almost exclusively through the nose during sleep. The researchers studied the resistance to the upper airway through either nasal or oral breathing and found that upper airway resistance during sleep and the propensity to obstructive sleep apnea are significantly lower while breathing nasally rather than orally.

Nasal obstruction during sleep results in mouth opening and mouth opening has been shown to increase the propensity to upper airway collapse. It has been shown that jaw opening is associated with posterior movement of the angle of the jaw, thus compromising the oropharyngeal airway diameter. This is caused by the shortening of the upper airway dilator muscles located between the mandible and the hyoid bone. In addition, jaw opening profoundly affects the diameter of the retroglossal airway.

The author has shown that there are two distinct sites of airway obstruction during sleep with oral breathing, when nasal breathing is not efficient.

The Board of Veterans' Appeals in a decision dated December 24, 2003, Citation Nr: 0336453, Docket No. 03-00 071A, concluded that sinusitis (upper airway obstruction) significantly contributes to sleep apnea:

> "While the record clearly supports a finding that the veteran suffers from sleep apnea, the record is equivocal regarding the effect that the veteran's service-connected sinusitis has on his sleeping disorder. In the opinion of the February 2001 VA examiner the veteran's sinusitis was not an obvious cause of the veteran's sleep apnea. Test

results appear to indicate that the veteran's sleep apnea is positional in nature, being twice as common in the supine position. However, a more recent medical opinion from his VA primary care physician indicates that the veteran's chronic sinusitis, if not the total cause, contributes significantly to his obstructive sleep apnea. In light of the above medical evidence showing a relationship between the veteran's chronic sinusitis and his sleep apnea, the Board determines that 38 C.F.R. § 3.102 (2003) should be applied in this case."

Sleep Apnea Secondary to Service-Connected PTSD

Veterans with PTSD have a higher prevalence of obstructive sleep apnea (OSA) than the general population. In a recent study, 47.6% of combat veterans with PTSD were found to have OSA compared to only 12.5% of healthy controls.

Scientists at the Madigan Army Medical Center have recently examined the incidence of sleep apnea in military personnel. In the study, *Sleep Disorders and Associated Medical Comorbidities in Active Duty Military Personnel*, Mysliwiec et al. observed that sleep disturbances are increasing in frequency and are commonly diagnosed during deployment and when military personnel return from deployment (redeployment). Recent evidence suggests the increased incidence of sleep disturbances in redeployed military personnel is potentially related to PTSD, depression, anxiety, or mTBI:

> "Medical comorbidities were frequently identified in military personnel undergoing PSG (sleep study), with 58.1% having one or more service-related illnesses. The percentages of military personnel with PTSD (13.2%) and mTBI (12.8%) are similar to previous reports, whereas a larger percentage of those in the study's study had depression (22.6%) and anxiety (16.8%)... Further, the sleep disturbances of insomnia and nightmares can persist despite appropriate therapy for PTSD..."

An estimated 26% to 31% of veterans in the U.S. are affected by PTSD in their lifetime. Individuals with PTSD often report sleep disturbances including trouble in falling and maintaining sleep, recurrent nightmares about trauma, and other disruptive nocturnal behaviors such as anxiety and night terrors during sleep.

Untreated OSA accentuates the sleep-related symptoms of PTSD, especially the number and intensity of nightmares, repeated awakenings, difficulty falling back to sleep, and increase in daytime sleepiness and tiredness. A growing body of evidence suggests that disturbed sleep is more likely to be a core feature of PTSD rather than just a secondary symptom.

Hypoxia, sympathetic discharge from respiratory disturbances, dysfunctional REM sleep and abnormal REM mechanism are proposed as a mechanism for sleep apnea in PTSD patients.

Dorland's Illustrated Medical Dictionary defines obstructive sleep apnea as sleep apnea resulting from collapse or obstruction of the airway with the inhibition of muscle tone that occurs during REM sleep. (Dorland. Dorland's Illustrated Medical Dictionary)

REM sleep is the period of sleep during which the brain waves are fast and of low voltage, and autonomic activities, such as heart rate and respiration, are irregular. This type of sleep is associated with dreaming, mild involuntary muscle jerks, and rapid eye movements (REM). It usually occurs three to four times each night at intervals of 80 to 120 minutes, each occurrence lasting from 5 minutes to more than an hour. In adults, about 20% of sleep is REM sleep and 80% is NREM (non–rapid eye movement) sleep. (Dorland. Dorland's Illustrated Medical Dictionary)

Kobayashi et al. conducted a meta-analytic review of 20 polysomnographic studies comparing sleep in people with and without PTSD. Results showed that PTSD patients had more stage 1 sleep, less slow wave sleep, and greater rapid-eye-movement density compared to people without PTSD.

A recent study showed that treatment of OSA with CPAP is associated with a decrease in the number of nightmares and daytime sleepiness in PTSD patients. This study also showed a positive correlation of REM sleep percentage with the number of nightmares. This supports the hypothesis that dysfunctional REM sleep mechanism may be involved in the pathogenesis of PTSD.

A recent study reported that REM, AHI and interrupted sleep at night were independent predictors of nightmares in OSA patients, and CPAP therapy results in significant improvement in nightmare occurrence. Apparently when a patient spends more time in REM the likelihood of having nightmares becomes higher. REM suppression with prazosin, an α-1 inhibitor, showed improvement in combat-related PTSD nightmares and sleep quality in active-duty soldiers in a recent trial. This may indicate that suppressing the "dysfunctional REM" in PTSD patients may have helped reduce symptoms. The subjective sleep disturbance in posttraumatic stress disorder (PTSD), including the repetitive, stereotypical anxiety dream, suggests dysfunctional rapid eye movement (REM) sleep mechanisms.

The polysomnograms (sleep study) of a group of physically healthy combat veterans with current PTSD were compared with those of an age-appropriate normal control group. Tonic and phasic REM sleep measures in the PTSD subjects were elevated on the second night of recorded sleep. Increased phasic REM sleep activity persisted in the PTSD group on the subsequent night. During the study, an anxiety dream occurred in a PTSD subject in REM sleep. The results are consistent with the view that a dysregulation of the REM sleep control system, particularly phasic event generation, may be involved in the pathogenesis of PTSD.

OSA patients were shown to maintain their upper airway patency in wakefulness via a compensatory, augmented EMG activity of their airway dilator muscles, during wakefulness [and non-rapid eye movement (NREM) sleep]. Remarkably, sleep apnea patients experience little or no problems with their breathing or airway patency while awake. In fact, the great majority of people with sleep apnea possess ventilatory control systems that are capable of precise regulation of their alveolar ventilation and arterial blood gases with extremely small variations from the norm.

Electrical activity from medullary inspiratory neurons, and EMG activity of diaphragm and abductor muscles of the upper airway in healthy humans show reductions in amplitude upon the transition from awake to NREM sleep, usually accompanied by a mild to moderate hypoventilation and two- to fivefold increases in upper airway resistance.

A fast and highly variable breathing frequency is a hallmark of rapid eye movement (REM) sleep in mammals. An excitatory drive to breathe is common in REM, with increased diaphragmatic EMG activity and increased activity in many medullary respiratory neurons above those levels observed in NREM sleep or quiet wakefulness. In REM sleep, there are both tonic excitatory inputs and phasic inhibitory inputs in the brain respiratory centers that account for irregularities in breathing pattern, as well as the loss of excitation, which contributes to hypotonia of the muscles of the upper airway. This results in collapse of the airway leading to sleep apnea.

In a recent decision by the Board of Veterans' Appeals (Docket No. 11-01922, March 28, 2016), the Board granted service connection for obstructive sleep apnea secondary to PTSD based on this author's IMO:

> "On September 2012 VA examination, the diagnosis was obstructive sleep apnea. The examiner reported that he found no valid medical literature to support the claim that sleep apnea is proximately due to or the result of PTSD. Therefore, the examiner opined that it was less likely as not the Veteran's sleep apnea was caused by or a result of his PTSD. A June 2014 letter from Dr. D. Anaise included an opinion that the Veteran's sleep apnea was more likely than not secondary to his service-connected PTSD. The letter cited medical literature as evidence in support of the opinion, and included such medical literature in support of the Veteran's claim. Such evidence was also in support of a causal relationship between sleep apnea and PTSD. The Board notes that the September 2012 VA opinion against the Veteran's claim cited the lack of medical literature in support of a causal relationship between PTSD and sleep apnea as a basis for concluding the Veteran's sleep apnea was less likely as not caused by or a result of his PTSD. In contrast, the June 2014 letter from Dr. D. Anaise indicated there was a significant volume of medical literature to support the Veteran's claim, and cited to such evidence in support of his opinion that the Veteran's obstructive sleep apnea was more likely than not secondary to his service-connected PTSD. The Board finds the June 2014 letter and opinion from

Dr. D. Anaise to be more probative and persuasive in this case as it was based on a review of the Veteran's treatment records, cited supporting medical literature, and was provided by a medical expert competent to provide an opinion as to the etiology of the Veteran's sleep apnea. Hence, entitlement to service connection for obstructive sleep apnea as secondary to service-connected PTSD is warranted."

Sleep Apnea Secondary to Chronic Pain Syndrome

Chronic pain and disrupted sleep are commonly associated and they share a clear cause-and-effect relationship.

A bi-directional relationship exists between pain and sleep disturbances. Pain fragments sleep continuity, impairs sleep quality, and disrupts normal sleep architecture. Reciprocally, poor quality or insufficient quality of sleep may decrease the pain threshold, impair recovery from injuries, or further exacerbate the pain response. Painful stimuli produce micro-arousals, which disrupt sleep continuity and alter normal sleep.

Chronic pain is associated with increased high frequency EEG activity and a decrease in slow frequency EEG activity. Furthermore, chronic pain is associated with the appearance of alpha waves superimposed on slower EEG frequencies, or "alpha-delta" sleep. In short, pain produces a state of shallow sleep while disrupting restorative slow-wave sleep.

An estimated 28 million Americans have sleep complaints due to chronic pain syndromes. Among patients with chronic pain, more than 50% experience sleep disturbances. Some reports show that as many as 70%-88% of patients with chronic pain report sleep trouble. Sleep disturbance shows an independent and linear correlation with pain severity, even after controlling for health measures and sleeping habits. Sleep complaints portend worse outcomes among those with chronic pain.

Mysliwiec et al. reported in the study *Sleep Disorders and Associated Medical Comorbidities in Active Duty Military Personnel*:

> "Military personnel with the diagnosis of pain syndromes were more likely to have insomnia. Poor sleep is a recognized symptom in individuals who have medical disorders associated with pain. Previous studies using both questionnaires and PSGs have reported patients with pain have difficulties initiating and maintaining sleep, supporting the association of pain syndromes with insomnia.[1] In the study's cohort, 24.7% were identified as taking medications for pain."

Pain causes sleep apnea in a manner similar to that discussed in sleep apnea in PTSD; namely by dysregulation of REM sleep. Moldofsky reported in *Sleep and pain* (Sleep Med Rev. 2001 Oct; 5(5):385-396) that painful disorders interfere with sleep.

Migraine and cluster headaches are related to REM sleep, whereas headache is associated with snoring and sleep apnea. The management of the sleep disorder ameliorates both morning headache and migraine. Noxious stimuli administered into muscles during slow-wave sleep (SWS) result in decreases in delta and sigma but an increase in alpha and beta EEG frequencies during sleep. Noise stimuli that disrupt SWS result in unrefreshing sleep, diffuse musculoskeletal pain, tenderness, and fatigue in normal healthy subjects.

Such symptoms accompany alpha EEG sleep patterns that often occur in patients with fibromyalgia. The alpha EEG patterns include phasic and tonic alpha EEG sleep as well as periodic K alpha EEG sleep or frequent periodic cyclical alternating pattern. Moreover, alpha EEG sleep, as well as sleep-related breathing disorder and periodic limb movement disorder, occur in some patients with fibromyalgia, rheumatoid arthritis and osteoarthritis. Depression and not alpha EEG sleep are features of somatoform pain disorder. Disturbances in sleep, pain, behavior and psychological distress influence return to work in workers who have suffered a soft tissue injury, e.g. low back pain. Patients with irritable bowel disorder have disturbed sleep and have increased REM sleep. In conclusion, there is a reciprocal relationship between sleep quality and pain.

Sleep Apnea Secondary to Narcotics Prescribed for Service-Connected Conditions

Narcotics, in particular opioids, have several effects on respiratory physiology, which are more pronounced during sleep. They decrease central respiratory patterns, respiratory rate, and tidal volume. They also increase airway resistance and decrease the patency of the upper airways. This may lead to ineffective ventilation and upper airway obstruction in susceptible individuals. These agents can produce irregularities in normal breathing patterns. Irregular respiratory pauses and gasping may lead to erratic breathing and significant variability in respiratory rate and effort. This ataxic breathing, is observed in the majority of patients with long-term opiate use.

A study of 71 patients with long-term methadone use found OSA in 35% of the patients. Although central sleep apnea (CSA) is classically associated with opioid use, it appears that OSA is more commonly encountered. Among patients receiving acute oral narcotics, OSA was observed in 35.2% of the patients and CSA in only 14.1%.

In a study assessing methadone maintenance patients with subjective sleep complaints, OSA was significantly more common than CSA. Similarly, OSA was diagnosed in 35%-57% of patients managed in long-term pain clinics. In an observational controlled trial of non-obese long-term opioid users, the majority of patients were found to have sleep-disordered breathing, with a mean apnea/hypopnea index of 43.9 ± 1.2. Most apneas were obstructive and not central events.

Alattar et al. studied the relation between medications prescribed for chronic pain and sleep apnea. Chronic pain patients on opioid therapy received overnight polysomnographies (sleep studies). The apnea-hypopnea index was abnormal (> or =5 per hour) in 75% of patients (39% had obstructive sleep apnea, 4% had sleep apnea of indeterminate type, 24% had central sleep apnea, and 8% had both central and obstructive sleep apnea).

Sleep Apnea Secondary to Service-Connected Tinnitus

Approximately 60% of patients with tinnitus experience disturbances of the normal sleep pattern.

German scientists performed polysomnography on 26 patients with tinnitus and sleep disturbances. In 17 of 26 patients, polysomnography revealed a pathological sleep analysis. 10 patients were diagnosed with obstructive sleep apnea syndrome, and 4 were diagnosed with insomnia and an increased index of arousals as well as a reduction of deep sleep and REM-phases. Pathological movements of the legs were seen in 3 cases. Six of 9 patients with normal sleep during the whole night displayed a prolonged latency period until falling asleep.

Sleep disturbance is a common and frequent complaint reported by tinnitus sufferers. Recent studies have shown that when insomnia and depression are associated with tinnitus there is decreased tolerance and increased discomfort with the tinnitus.

The apparent cause of sleep apnea in patients suffering from tinnitus is the disruption of sleep patterns, specifically disruption of rapid eye movement (REM).

OSA patients were shown to maintain their upper airway patency in wakefulness via a compensatory, augmented EMG activity of their airway dilator muscles, during wakefulness [and non-rapid eye movement (NREM) sleep]. Remarkably, sleep apnea patients experience little or no problems with their breathing or airway patency while awake. In fact, the great majority of people with sleep apnea possess ventilatory control systems that are capable of precise regulation of their alveolar ventilation and arterial blood gases with extremely small variations from the norm.

Electrical activity from medullary inspiratory neurons, and EMG activity of diaphragm and abductor muscles of the upper airway in healthy humans show reductions in amplitude upon the transition from awake to NREM sleep, usually accompanied by a mild to moderate hypoventilation and two- to fivefold increases in upper airway resistance.

A fast and highly variable breathing frequency is a hallmark of rapid eye movement (REM) sleep in mammals. An excitatory drive to breathe is common in REM, with increased diaphragmatic EMG activity and increased activity in many medullary respiratory neurons above those levels observed in NREM sleep or quiet wakefulness. In REM sleep, there are both tonic excitatory inputs and phasic inhibitory inputs in the brain respiratory centers that account for irregularities in breathing pattern, as well as the loss of excitation, which contributes to hypotonia of the muscles of the upper airway. This results in collapse of the airway leading to sleep apnea.

In a recent study, scientists observed:

> "All tinnitus patients had a statistically significant alteration in sleep stages. Average percentage of stage 1 + stage 2 was 85.4% ± 6.3, whereas, in the control group, the average percentage of stage 1 + stage 2 was 54.9 ± 11.2 ($p < 0.001$). Stages 3 and 4 and rapid eye movement (REM) sleep was lacking in all tinnitus patients with an average percentage of 6.4 ± 4.9 of REM sleep, and 6.4 ± 4.9 of stages 3 + 4. The control group showed an average percentage of 21.5 ± 3.6 of REM sleep and 21.5 ± 3.6 of stages 3 + 4 ($p < 0.001$)."

Quantitative non-rapid eye movement sleep analysis revealed lower spectral power in the delta frequency band in the tinnitus group compared to controls, and this decrease was correlated with subjective sleep complaints (the lower the delta spectral power, the greater the complaints).

Sleep Apnea Secondary to Service-Connected Chronic Obstructive Airway Disease (COPD) or Asthma

Several studies have confirmed that asthmatic patients are more prone to develop OSA symptoms than are members of the general population. The common asthmatic features that promote OSAS symptoms are nasal obstruction, a decrease in pharyngeal cross sectional area, and an increase in upper airway collapsibility (Alkhalil, M.; Schulman, E.; Getsy, J. *Obstructive Sleep Apnea Syndrome and Asthma: What Are the Links?* J Clin Sleep Med 2009;5(l):71-78).

The August 2007 National Asthma Education and Prevention Program Expert Panel Report 3 (EPR3) recommended that clinicians evaluate symptoms that suggest OSAS in unstable, poorly controlled asthmatic patients. Patients with OSAS have an increased vagal tone during sleep as a consequence of partial or complete airway obstruction occurring during apneas. The mechanics of this potent vagal stimulation are similar to those of the Muller maneuver, which consists of an inspiratory effort against a closed glottis. Increased vagal tone occurring during apnea episodes could be a trigger for nocturnal asthma attacks in sleep apnea patients (Morrison, J.F.; Pearson, S.B.; Dean H.G. *Parasympathetic nervous system in nocturnal asthma.* BMJ. 1988;296:1427-9).

In fact, several studies have shown that increased vagal tone stimulates the muscarinic receptors located in the central airways leading to bronchoconstriction and causing nocturnal asthma. Furthermore, suppression of the increased vagal tone by inhaled anticholinergic drugs leads to improvement in forced expiratory flow, reduction in early morning falls in peak expiratory flow, and protection against nocturnal asthma symptoms (Coe C.I.; Barnes P.J. *Reduction of nocturnal asthma by an inhaled anticholinergic drug*, Chest. 1986;90:485-8).

Another factor in the neural reflex mechanism involves the neural receptors at the glottic inlets and in the laryngeal region; these receptors have powerful reflex Broncho constrictive activity. Nadal et al. showed that mechanical irritation of the laryngeal mucosa increased total lung resistance distal to the larynx (Nadel J.A.; Widdicombe J.G. *Reflex effects of upper airway irritation on total lung resistance and blood pressure* J Appl Physiol. 1962;17:861-5.)The BVA has held that OSA is secondary to asthma (Docket No. 11-08 722, February 8, 2016) based on this author's IMO:

> "The Veteran seeks service connection for asthma and sleep apnea...
>
> The VHA physician stated that it was less likely than not that sleep apnea had its onset during service. He noted that asthma has been noted to be associated with increased risk of developing obstructive sleep apnea in some epidemiological studies, but that the nature of the association between the two conditions is not fully understood...
>
> The Veteran's attorney, who is a physician, provided a statement that related the Veteran's sleep apnea to his asthma. This statement cited

medical literature in support of this conclusion and provided a description of the process by which asthma can result in sleep apnea.

The Board finds that the medical evidence for and against the claim is at least in relative equipoise. Resolving reasonable doubt in favor of the Veteran, there is a basis of entitlement to service connection on a secondary basis under 38 C.F.R. § 3.310. See 38 U.S.C.A. § 5107(b); 38 C.F.R. § 3.102."

In the same case, I also argued successfully that Veteran is entitled to have separate disability ratings for asthma and OSA, rather than a combined rating. The VA claimed that sleep apnea and asthma deserve one rating as both conditions involve the lung:

"This statement is incorrect. Asthma is a lung disease which is caused by constriction of the small bronchi. Obstructive sleep apnea is a condition that causes collapse of the major airway in the neck it does not involve the lung directly, and thus, it is totally a separate medical condition.

OSA is caused by soft tissue collapse in the pharynx not the lung. OSA patients were shown to maintain their upper airway patency in wakefulness via a compensatory, augmented EMG activity of their airway dilator muscles, which extended an earlier report of more frequently occurring genioglossus EMG activity during wakefulness [and non-rapid eye movement (NREM) sleep] in OSA patients. Remarkably, sleep apnea patients experience little or no problems with their breathing or airway patency while awake. In fact, the great majority of people with sleep apnea possess ventilatory control systems that are capable of precise regulation of their alveolar ventilation and arterial blood gases with extremely small variations from the norm.

It is, thus, a mistake to attribute obstructive sleep apnea to a lung disease. It is a failure of the upper airway in response to derangement of brain function, and thus, obstructive sleep apnea is not a disease of the lung.

In *Esteban v. Brown* No. 92-693 the Court allowed for separate ratings where the symptomatology for one condition was not duplicative of or overlapping with the symptomatology of the other."

Sleep Apnea Secondary to Service-Connected Gastroesophageal Reflux Disease (GERD)

GERD occurs in up to 60% of OSA patients; comparatively, it occurs in only 20% of the general population. Several studies showed that OSA was more common in GERD patients than in the general population.

Several observations suggest close causative relationship between GERD and OSA. Nasal continuous positive airway pressure treatment for OSA improves the symptoms of GERD. Proton pump inhibitor treatment reduces the obstructive events and improves the apnea hypopnea index in OSA patients.

Several mechanisms have been suggested to explain why patients suffering from GERD develop OSA. The connection between the diaphragm and lower esophageal sphincter through the phrenoesophageal ligament is considered the mechanism of GERD in OSA patients.

Many patients with GERD have nocturnal re-flux symptoms, because sleep itself leads to proximal migration of gastric acid and aspiration into the tracheal-bronchial tree. The proximal migration of refluxed gastric contents and micro aspiration of acid during sleep can cause inflammation and edema of the upper airway, as well as bronchoconstriction, thereby predisposing to OSA. The refluxed gastric acid in the distal esophagus in GERD also triggers a vagal reflex that can facilitate bronchospasm.

Nocturnal GERD is considered to have a greater risk for respiratory complications including OSA. According to previous studies, nocturnal symptoms of GERD are more common in patients with OSA and may be improved by treatment with nasal continuous positive airway pressure. A recent study also showed that having persistent nocturnal symptoms of GERD is linked to recent development of OSA symptoms.

Sleep Apnea and Obesity

Obesity is a common cause of OSA. Yet, the perception that fat deposition in the neck is the cause of airway obstruction in sleep apnea is incorrect.

Central, or visceral, obesity is associated with the greatest risk for OSA. This suggests that factors other than pure mechanical load may contribute to the pathogenesis of respiratory disturbances during sleep. Visceral fat depots, which represent a rich source of humoral mediators and inflammatory cytokines, can impact on neural pathways associated with respiratory control.

Perhaps the most well-studied adipocyte (fat cell) - derived factor affecting respiratory control is leptin, which was initially determined to have a primary role of binding to receptors in the hypothalamus to reduce satiety and increase metabolism. Leptin, a hormone secreted by fat cells, can also act as a respiratory stimulant, and impairment of the leptin signaling pathway, is associated with obesity hypoventilation syndrome in humans. Leptin plays a role in nocturnal hypoventilation, particularly in REM sleep where respiration is markedly depressed in leptin-deficient mice.

Visceral adipose tissue releases many other humoral factors including classical proinflammatory cytokines such as tumor necrosis factor-α (TNF-α) and interleukin (IL)-6 that are elevated in OSA and can be reduced with

CPAP therapy. These and other proinflammatory cytokines may impact on sleep.

Insulin resistance is the hallmark symptom of the metabolic syndrome. The metabolic syndrome has many features in common with OSA including obesity, hyperlipidemia, hypertension, and insulin resistance. OSA is so interwoven in the fabric of the metabolic syndrome, or Syndrome X, that the combination of OSA and metabolic syndrome has been labeled "Syndrome Z" (Wilcox I, McNamara SG, Collins FL, Grunstein RR, Sullivan CE. "Syndrome Z": the interaction of sleep apnea, vascular risk factors and heart disease. Thorax 53 Suppl 3: S25–S28, 1998).

The development of insulin resistance and type 2 diabetes is largely dependent on the presence of obesity. There is now a growing body of evidence that the "lipotoxic" effects of obesity play an important role in the pathogenesis of insulin resistance. Supporting this hypothesis are observations that acute hyperlipidemia induces insulin resistance and that decreasing the metabolic availability of lipids in vivo increases insulin sensitivity.

Adipocytes are a major source of circulating cytokines that both induce and respond to proinflammatory stress pathways. In general, cytokines are secreted into the circulation as a function of the size of an adipocyte, consequently establishing a positive relationship between adiposity and circulating cytokines.

For example, two important inflammatory cytokines, TNF-α and IL-6, have elevated circulating levels in obesity and are decreased by weight loss. Clinical studies suggest that OSA may have an independent role in further increasing circulating levels of TNF-α, IL-6, as well as the general inflammatory marker C-reactive protein, above the levels seen in obese, non-apneic control subjects, as well as in OSA patients treated with CPAP (Minoguchi K, Tazaki T, Yokoe T, Minoguchi H, Watanabe Y, Yamamoto M, Adachi M. Elevated production of tumor necrosis factor-alpha by monocytes in patients with obstructive sleep apnea syndrome. Chest 126: 1473–1479, 2004).

Sleep Apnea Secondary to Service-Connected Diabetes Mellitus

There is a high prevalence of obstructive sleep apnea in people with type 2 diabetes and abnormal glucose metabolism.

The International Diabetes Federation (IDF) Taskforce on Epidemiology and Prevention convened a Working Group in February 2007 to review the effect of diabetes on OSA. Polysomnography testing showed OSA in up to 9% of women and 24% of men with diabetes. There has long been a recognized association between type 2 diabetes and OSA, and there is emerging evidence that this relationship is likely to be at least partially independent of adiposity. Cross-sectional estimates from clinic populations and population studies suggest that up to 40% of patients with OSA will have diabetes.

Two large studies with clinic-based sample sizes of 250–300 subjects both demonstrated a positive association, independent of obesity, between the severity of OSA and indexes of insulin resistance determined by fasting insulin and glucose. Insulin resistance is a central part of the metabolic syndrome. The metabolic syndrome has many features in common with OSA including obesity, hyperlipidemia, hypertension and insulin resistance. OSA is so interwoven in the fabric of the metabolic syndrome, or Syndrome X, that the combination of OSA and metabolic syndrome has been labeled "Syndrome Z."

Scientists reported that the pro-inflammatory cytokines interleukin-6 (IL-6) and tumor necrosis factor-alpha (TNFalpha) were elevated in patients with disorders of excessive daytime sleepiness (EDS) and proposed that these cytokines were mediators of daytime sleepiness. They also reported that IL-6, TNFalpha, and insulin levels were elevated in sleep apnea independently of obesity.

The prevalence of metabolic syndrome in the US population, from the Third National Health and Nutrition Examination Survey (1988-1994), parallels the prevalence of symptomatic sleep apnea. This supports the hypothesis that cytokines and insulin resistance are mediators of EDS and sleep apnea in humans.

Sleep Apnea Secondary to Service-Connected Stroke and Ischemic Heart Disease

Obstructive sleep apnea (OSA) is characterized by repetitive interruption of ventilation during sleep caused by collapse of the pharyngeal airway. A recent meta-analysis that combined the results from nine prospective cohort studies reported that OSA was significantly associated with stroke in participants without previous cardiovascular disease.

Compared with the general population, patients with stroke or ischemic heart disease (IHD) have 3 to 4 times higher prevalence of OSA, approximately 60% to 70%. Stern, et al. found that OSA is present in up to 72% of ischemic and hemorrhagic stroke and TIA patients. The OSA was primarily obstructive in nature, with only 7% of patients having primarily central apneas. The OSA frequency was high in stroke patients despite a relatively low average BMI of 26.4 kg/m^2.

It is most likely that the cause of sleep apnea in stroke victims is aberration in REM sleep. In *Causes of Excessive Daytime Sleepiness in Patients with Acute Stroke-A Polysomnographic Study*, Klobučníková et al. reported that sleep disorders are common in stroke patients. Sleep-disordered breathing (SDB), which is present in up to 72% of stroke patients, is the most frequent cause of excessive daytime sleepiness (EDS) in the common population. 102 patients with the clinical diagnosis of acute stroke were enrolled into the study. EDS was present in 21 patients (20.6%). It was found that in a population with EDS, there is a significantly higher number of obstructive apneic pauses, central apneic pauses, as well as significantly higher values of respiratory disturbance index (RDI), RDI during non-rapid eye movement sleep, desaturation index, and significant decrease of REM sleep duration.

Sleep Apnea Secondary to Service-Connected Cervical Spine Abnormalities

Patients with cervical spine abnormalities secondary to spondyloarthropathy or rheumatoid arthritis are known to have a very high incidence of obstructive sleep apnea. Sleep apnea is a risk factor for high mortality of rheumatoid arthritis (RA) patients.

In the research article, *Sleep apnea in rheumatoid arthritis patients with occipitocervical lesions: the prevalence and associated radiographic features*, Naoki Shoda et al. examined the prevalence of sleep apnea in RA patients with cervical lesions. Twenty-nine RA patients requiring surgery for progressive myelopathy due to occipito-cervical lesions were preoperatively evaluated. Twenty-three (79%) had sleep apnea, and all of them were classified as the obstructive type. The authors observed that:

> "Obstructive sleep apnea was caused by the reduction of the airway space which is determined by an interaction between mechanical properties of the airway itself and neurological regulations of the dilator muscles."

They suggested that both mechanisms could possibly be affected by RA with cervical lesions. First, the decrease of cervical length may give rise to a bending force and horizontal pressure on the soft tissues surrounding the airway, which, in turn, may cause the mechanical compression of the airway. Secondly, the vertical translocation caused by the RA occipitocervical lesions may "lead to compression of cranial nerves V, VII, IX, X, XII that are known to control the airway dilator muscles. The neurological dysfunction of the muscles may cause the collapse of the airway."

Similarly, it has been proposed that spondyloarthrosis patients are at increased risk for OSA because of structural changes in the cervical spine. This hypothesis is supported by reports of improvement in OSA after surgical removal of excessively bulky, pathologic bone from the anterior cervical spine.

OSA has also been shown to be caused by anterior cervical spine fusion and the insertion of a plate. In the study, *Anterior cervical spine fusion and sleep disordered breathing*, Guilleminault et al. reviewed 12 patients who developed OSA in association with anterior cervical spine fusion. Four subsequent patients were studied prospectively before C2 to C4 anterior fusion and documented to have OSA by questionnaire, visual analogue scales, polysomnography, and multiple sleep latency tests. The authors found that placement of the anterior cervical plates reduced the size of the upper airway. Symptoms and objective findings were controlled with nasal continuous positive airway pressure.

In addition, Krieger et al. reported cases of sleep apnea following spinal surgery in the Journal of Neurosurgery, *Sleep-induced apnea 2. Respiratory failure after anterior spinal surgery* (Journal of Neurosurgery, 1974 Feb; 40(2):181-5).

Migraines Secondary to Service-Connected Sleep Apnea

Hildegard Hidalgo, MD, from the Department of Neurology at Kamillus-Klinik in Asbach, Germany reported that 25% of patients with OSA also have migraines. In this prospective study, the researchers investigated the possible role of hypoxia during sleep and the long-term effects of CPAP therapy on migraine. They screened 314 potential participants with OSA. The participants had a mean Epworth Sleepiness Scale score of 9.8 ± 4.8 and a mean AHI of 27.4 ± 25.4 episodes/hour at baseline. Twenty-one had migraine with aura, 19 had migraine without aura, and 1 had chronic migraine. Thirty patients accepted CPAP therapy. Compared with baseline, polysomnography showed significant improvements at 1 year in AHI, mean duration of sleep-related breathing disorders, oxygen desaturation index (all $P < .001$), arousal index ($P < .002$), slow wave sleep ($P = .031$), and other measures. CPAP therapy significantly reduced migraine measures and disease burden.

Hypertension Secondary to Service-Connected Sleep Apnea

A recent large multicenter study, *"Elevated nocturnal and morning blood pressure in patients with obstructive sleep apnea syndrome,"* by Dr. He et al. found an excellent correlation between high blood pressure and obstructive sleep apnea after analysis of findings from 20 teaching hospitals, included 2297 patients. The study concluded "OSA may result in higher BP levels at all four time points [daytime, nighttime, evening and morning]. The ratios of nighttime/daytime and morning/evening BP increase with increased AHI [apnea-hypopnea index]."

Sleep Apnea Secondary to Service-Connected Fibromyalgia

Disordered sleep is such a prominent symptom in fibromyalgia that the American College of Rheumatology included symptoms such as waking unrefreshed, fatigue, tiredness, and insomnia in the 2010 diagnostic criteria for fibromyalgia.

Togo et al. evaluated polysomnograms of chronic fatigue syndrome (CFS) patients with and without fibromyalgia to determine whether patients in either group had elevated rates of sleep-disturbed breathing (obstructive sleep apnea or upper airway resistance syndrome) or periodic leg movement disorder. They also looked at whether feelings of unrefreshing sleep were associated with differences in sleep architecture from normal. They reported that CFS patients had significant differences in polysomnographic findings from healthy controls, and felt sleepier and more fatigued than controls after a night's sleep. CFS patients as a group had less total sleep time, lower sleep efficiency, and less rapid eye movement sleep than controls. This sleep disruption may explain the overwhelming fatigue, report of unrefreshing sleep, and pain in this subgroup of patients.

The Association between fibromyalgia and upper airway resistance syndrome was studied by Gold et al. They studied twenty-eight women with fibromyalgia diagnosed by rheumatologists using established criteria. Eighteen of the 28 women with fibromyalgia and all the women with UARS underwent a full-night polysomnogram. All participants also had a nasal continuous positive airway pressure (CPAP) study. Twenty-seven of the twenty-eight women with fibromyalgia had sleep-disordered breathing. The pharyngeal critical pressure of the patients with fibromyalgia was -6.5 +/- 3.5 cmH2O (mean +/- SD) compared to -5.8 +/- 3.5 cmH2O for patients with UARS (P = .62). Treatment of 14 consecutive patients with nasal CPAP resulted in an improvement in functional symptoms. The researchers concluded:

> "Inspiratory airflow limitation is a common inspiratory airflow pattern during sleep in women with fibromyalgia. Our findings are compatible with the hypothesis that inspiratory flow limitation during sleep plays a role in the development of the functional somatic syndromes."

Upper Airway Resistance Syndrome (UARS)

The upper airway resistance syndrome (UARS) is a recently described form of sleep-disordered breathing in which repetitive increases in resistance to airflow within the upper airway lead to brief arousals and daytime somnolence.

The primary symptom of daytime somnolence appears to result directly from repetitive EEG arousals. Aside from daytime somnolence, hypertension is an important sequelae of this disorder, likely resulting from autonomic and cardiovascular changes induced by increased negative intrathoracic pressure. Nasal continuous positive airway pressure is the most efficacious form of therapy.

A report, *Upper Airway Resistance Syndrome*, from the Ohio Sleep Medicine Institute describes how upper airway resistance syndrome manifests itself; initially with snoring which then progresses to full-blown obstructive sleep apnea associated with non-refreshing sleep, and excessive daytime sleepiness. The authors concluded, "we now believe that UARS represents a progression of disease bridging the transition from "benign snoring" to obstructive sleep apnea."

During sleep the muscles of the airway become relaxed. The relaxation of these muscles in turn reduces the diameter of the airway. Typically, the airway of a person with UARS is already restricted or reduced in size, and this natural relaxation reduces the airway diameter further. Therefore, breathing becomes labored. It can be likened to breathing through a straw.

The pathophysiology of UARS is similar to that of obstructive sleep apnea/hypopnea syndrome in that abnormal upper airway resistance during sleep leads to unwanted physiologic consequences. Increased upper airway resistance in this disorder does not lead to cessation of airflow (apnea) or decrease in airflow (hypopnea), but instead leads to an arousal secondary to increased work of breathing to overcome the resistance. Repeated and multiple arousals (of which the person is usually unaware) result in an abnormal sleep architecture and daytime somnolence (sleepiness). Arousals result in sympathetic activation, and UARS is therefore likely to cause hypertension similar to obstructive sleep apnea syndrome. (This has not been verified in large clinical populations because of the relatively small number of people with UARS in the larger epidemiologic studies so far. However, repeated arousals in individuals have clearly shown relation to sympathetic activation and elevation in blood pressure.)

Treatment for UARS is essentially the same as that for obstructive sleep apnea.

Sleep Apnea Caused by Antidepressants

In a large study (1779 patients) from the University of Queensland, *Associations Between the Use of Common Medications and Sleep Architecture in Patients with Untreated Obstructive Sleep Apnea*, researchers found a strong association between the use of antidepressant medications like Sertaline/Zoloft and sleep apnea. Consistent associations with sleep-architecture measures were found for SSRI (paroxetine/fluoxetine and sertraline).

These effects were found after controlling for variables such as age, BMI, RDI, and sex. Specifically, an association between a lower percentage of REM sleep was found in patients who were taking paroxetine/fluoxetine or sertraline (about 7% lower), compared with those not taking any medications.

Nicholson and Pascoe have reported that fluoxetine decreased sleep efficiency and total sleep time and increased awakenings in healthy adults. The finding of lower sleep efficiency in patients taking antidepressants is also consistent with previous reports that some SSRI antidepressant or anxiolytic medications can reduce sleep continuity.

Narcolepsy

Narcolepsy affects at least 2 in 1000 individuals.

Narcolepsy includes a tetrad of excessive sleepiness, cataplexy (sudden loss of muscle tone while awake, resulting in brief inability to move), sleep paralysis, and hypnagogic hallucinations. The full tetrad occurs in approximately 1 of 5000 people.

Narcolepsy is a disorder of rapid eye movement (REM) sleep regulation caused by disordered hypocretin neurotransmission, likely resulting from an autoimmune loss of hypocretin neurons in the lateral hypothalamus. The daytime symptoms of narcolepsy are accompanied by the intrusion of REM sleep into wakefulness.

Cataplexy is characterized by brief (seconds to a few minutes) loss of muscle tone (i.e., intrusion of REM atonia) triggered by emotions, most commonly laughter but also elation, surprise, and fear. If severe, the patient may fall. With milder attacks, a head nod or slurred speech can occur. Hypnagogic hallucinations that are vivid and dreamlike and that occur at sleep onset are more specific for narcolepsy than hypnopompic (i.e., sleep offset) hallucinations.

Sleep paralysis is the frightening experience of inability to move while aware, usually on awakening.

In addition to the tetrad, patients frequently have episodes of automatic behaviors with no recall, which can resemble complex partial seizures. Nocturnal sleep is often fragmented by frequent arousals, vivid dreams, or leg movements.

Sleep Apnea and Interstitial Lung Disease

The interstitial lung diseases (ILD) are a heterogeneous group of disorders characterized by varying degrees of fibrosis and inflammation of lung parenchyma. Sufferers exhibit lung restriction and exercise intolerance, often developing progressive hypoxia over time. Independent of the presence of daytime hypoxia, many individuals with ILD are observed to desaturate during sleep, with or without associated apnea.

There is mounting evidence that nocturnal hypoxia and sleep-disordered breathing (SDB) may contribute to adverse outcomes. Aside from resulting in poor sleep quality and daytime fatigue, transient repetitive desaturation and associated sympathetic nervous system activation may play a role in the development of pulmonary hypertension and contribute to increased mortality.

Not surprisingly, sleep quality is comparatively poorer than that of the normal population. Nocturnal cough, medications, breathing difficulties, hypoxia and obstructive apneas have all been implicated in disrupting sleep in this population. In 1985, Perez-Padilla et al. compared 11 ILD patients with age- and sex-matched controls. They reported decreased amounts of rapid eye movement (REM) sleep as well as significant sleep fragmentation in the patient group. Further prospective studies, with particular focus on Idiopathic Pulmonary Fibrosis (IPF) confirm these findings, and also report increased stage 1 and 2 sleep, reduced slow wave sleep and poorer overall sleep efficiency.

Patients with interstitial lung disease commonly exhibit abnormal sleep architecture and increased sleep fragmentation on polysomnography. Fatigue is a frequent complaint, and it is likely that poor sleep quality is a significant contributor.

A number of studies have shown that sleep disordered breathing is prevalent in this population, particularly in the idiopathic pulmonary fibrosis subgroup. The factors that predispose these patients to obstructive sleep apnea are not well understood. However, it is believed that reduced caudal traction on the upper airway can enhance collapsibility.

Ventilatory control system instability may also be an important factor, particularly in those with increased chemo-responsiveness, and in hypoxic conditions. Transient, repetitive nocturnal oxygen desaturation is frequently observed in interstitial lung disease, both with and without associated obstructive apneas. There is increasing evidence that sleep-desaturation is associated with increased mortality, and may be important in the pathogenesis of pulmonary hypertension in this population.

Sleep Apnea and Cardiovascular Disease (CVD)

Sleep apnea is associated with a variety of cardiovascular conditions ranging from hypertension to heart failure. OSA has become increasingly considered as a potential therapeutic target for either primary or secondary prevention of CVD.

OSA has been definitively shown to be an independent risk factor for the development of hypertension. Patients with mild to moderate OSA (AHI 5-14.9) were twice as likely to develop hypertension as were those without OSA. The odds ratio rose to 2.89 in patients with severe OSA (AHI > 15). Recent guidelines recommend screening for the presence of OSA in patients with refractory hypertension.

In one cross-sectional study, OSA was associated with a range of manifestations of CVD (stroke, heart failure, ischemic heart disease). The prevalence of CVD increased progressively with increasing AHI, with multivariable- adjusted relative odds (95% CI) of prevalent CVD for the second, third, and fourth quartiles of the AHI (versus the first) of 0.98 (0.77-1.24), 1.28 (1.02-1.61), and 1.42 (1.13-1.78), respectively.

Other studies show that OSA is associated with myocardial infarction and in those with known coronary disease. Patients with OSA have an increased risk of cardiovascular events and death. Cardiac arrhythmias and sudden cardiac death have also been shown to be more common in patients with OSA.

A variety of mechanisms and pathways may promote the development of CVD in those with OSA:

- Mechanical changes

  With each apneic or hypopneic episode, there is exaggerated negative pleural pressure. This may impact upon cardiac performance and induce shear stress on the vasculature.

- Intermittent hypoxia and oxidative stress

  Hypoxia is a strong stimulus for acute elevation of blood pressure. In chronic hypoxia and hypercarbia, chemoreceptors may undergo long-term adaptation and play a major role in elevating baseline blood pressure. In the short-term, both chemoreceptor and sympathetically activated processes may mediate the increases in blood pressure associated with simulated or spontaneous apneas.

  Evidence suggests that recurrent intermittent hypoxia-reoxygenation in OSA may lead to a state of oxidative stress and activation of inflammatory transcription pathways.

- Systemic inflammation, vasoactive mediators, and endothelial dysfunction

  Adverse changes in circulating levels of many vasoactive or inflammatory mediators including nitric oxide, interleukin-6, tumor necrosis factor, C-reactive protein, and platelet activation and coagulation factors have been described in OSA.

- Sympathetic activation

    Repeated oscillations in blood pressure following breathing events in OSA may reset central baroreceptors making them less sensitive, thus leading to persistent elevation of blood pressure. Furthermore, OSA increases catecholamine levels, which may increase the risk of CVD events and heart failure.

- Effects on lipids

    Evidence of contribution of OSA towards modification of circulating levels of lipids is conflicting. Animal studies have shown that intermittent hypoxia regulates genes of lipid biosynthesis, and that dyslipidemia and lipid peroxidation are dependent on the severity of the hypoxia. Both increased levels of oxidized LDL, and dysfunction of HDL have been described in OSA.

Sleep Apnea and Headaches/Migraines

Sleep-related symptoms are associated with painful conditions, partly because pain may interfere with sleep and vice versa. This dual cause and effect relationship has been known for many years through clinical experience with headache patients. The scientific literature addressing comorbidity of headache and sleep disturbances is growing.

Many epidemiological studies have evaluated the association with sleep apnea to nonspecific headache diagnoses (e.g. headache, morning headache, chronic daily headache), whereas relatively few epidemiological studies have focused on the specific diagnosis of tension-type headache (TTH). TTH is associated with sleep disorders, and subjects with TTH often report sleep complaints related to insomnia.

The impact of sleep complaints in migraineurs has been studied more extensively. Migraine is associated with several sleep problems, and this observation is supported by polysomnographic findings. Also, excess of sleep, insufficient sleep duration, and poor sleep quality are common triggering factors for migraine attacks.

According to a study from Sweden, severe sleep disturbance were five times more likely among migraineurs, and three times more likely among subjects with TTH. Other studies using different types of questionnaires have also reported a higher prevalence of sleep disturbances among migraineur and subjects with TTH, respectively. Studies have reported a higher prevalence of daytime sleepiness among migraineurs and insomnia among subjects with TTH.

A study found that the association between headache and severe sleep disturbance increased markedly in relation to the headache frequency. In accordance with other studies, the prevalence of sleep disturbances increased with higher frequency of headache/days per month and that subjects with chronic headache had more sleep disturbances compared with subjects with episodic headaches.

CHAPTER 5 - ORTHOPEDICS

Posttraumatic Osteoarthritis

Medical research clearly shows that soldiers are especially susceptible to osteoarthritis after discharge from the service, and that osteoarthritis may manifest itself many years after the initial injury. In addition, due to gait issues, an affected limb can result in the development of osteoarthritis in proximal joints.

Scientists from the San Antonio Military Medical Center and the United States Army Institute of surgical research have recently reviewed the incidence and severity of osteoarthritis in veterans serving in Iraq and Afghanistan, *Posttraumatic Osteoarthritis Caused by Battlefield Injuries: The Primary Source of Disability in Warriors*. Arthritis was recognized as a disabling condition an average of 19 ± 10 months after injury.

Brown et al. estimated that 12% of symptomatic OA is attributable to posttraumatic osteoarthritis (PTOA) of the hip, knee, or ankle. OA is the most common cause of disability among service members who are medically separated from active duty. Among those with osteoarthritis as an unfitting condition, injuries to the spine and shoulder occurred most commonly. The rate of arthritis by injured anatomic region varied considerably. Injuries to the knee resulted in OA in all cases, and the elbow and ankle joints became arthritic following injury in greater than 90% of cases. Traumatic injury was the cause of 94.4% of all cases of joint OA and 75% of cases of spine OA.

PTOA is a common and disabling condition in combat-wounded warriors. The prevalence of OA was 28% in the veteran study population, compared with 12% in the civilian trauma population. In veterans, the permanent disability resulting from combat-related traumatic arthritis is substantial. The diagnosis of arthritis is accelerated in this group, with an average time of <2 years from injury to determination of disability as a result of arthritis. PTOA affects not only the appendicular joints but is disabling following injury to the spine, as well.

Dominick et al. reported that U.S. veterans experience a higher frequency of OA, chronic joint symptoms, and activity limitations than do persons in the general population. The study shows that osteoarthritis in veterans is a result of wear and tear caused by excessive trauma to joints in the process of active military training and combat. The study is limited by the lack of follow-up, as the focus was solely on veterans of the recent conflict in the Middle East. Studies of veterans of the Vietnam and Korean conflicts clearly show that osteoarthritis occurs many years after discharge from the military service.

In a study published at the MSMR, a publication of the Armed Forces Health Surveillance Center (Volume 17, Number 12, December 2010), the investigators found that over the last 10 years 68,449 incident diagnosis of osteoarthritis and 43,254 incident diagnoses of spondylosis were identified. The incidence rate of osteoarthritis increased dramatically, by 65% from 2001 to 2006. The scientists concluded that military training and operational service activities are often physically demanding and sometimes traumatic, e.g. heavy load bearing, and hand-to-hand combat training. Musculoskeletal disorders including osteoarthritis have been associated with specific occupations and some military occupations are inherently stressful to bones and joints, including pilots and paratroopers.

The recent study from the Department of Veterans' Affairs explains why osteoarthritis appears many years after trauma to the joints, challenging long-held notions that osteoarthritis is a result mainly of wear and tear on the joints. Researchers led by Dr. William H. Robinson of the Department of Veterans' Affairs Palo Alto Health Care System and Stanford University have provided new insights into the immune-system changes that may trigger cartilage breakdown. Their report appears in the Nov. 6, 2011 online edition of Nature Medicine. "This research can lead to a better quality of life for Veterans and others with osteoarthritis," said Secretary of Veterans Affairs Eric K. Shinseki. "This is an example of how VA's research program can lead to many significant breakthroughs in health care." The researchers discovered that one component of the complement system, called the membrane attack complex, or MAC, is formed and activated in the joints of both humans and mice affected by osteoarthritis. They believe that when the MAC is aberrantly activated in the joints (a phenomenon called "dysregulation"), it induces low-grade inflammation and the production of enzymes that break down cartilage and result in the development of osteoarthritis.

This new study showed that initial damage to the joint sets in motion a chain of molecular events that escalates into an attack upon the damaged joint by one of the body's key defense systems against bacterial and viral infections, the so-called complement system. This sequence of events involves activation of a chain reaction called the "complement cascade," and begins early in the development of osteoarthritis. The complement system consists of an orchestra of proteins present in blood. Upon activation of the complement cascade — typically, in response to the presence of bacterial or viral infection — these proteins engage in a complex interplay, variously enhancing or inhibiting one another's actions at certain points and culminating in the activation of a protein cluster called the MAC (for "membrane attack complex"). By punching holes in the membranes of bacterial or virally infected human cells, the MAC helps to clear the body of infections.

Osteoarthritis is a degenerative disease of the discs and joints that affects millions of people worldwide. A third of people ages 60 and above suffer from the disease that causes pain and stiffness in hands, necks, knees and other joints. The VA estimates that more than 6 million World War II and Korean War Veterans are still living and could be affected. The finding may offer new insight into potential treatment. "Right now," Robinson says, "we don't have anything to offer osteoarthritis patients to treat their underlying disease. It would be incredible to find a way to slow it down."

The scientific literature also supports the finding that injury to one limb will result in osteoarthritis of proximal joints. Adriacchi hypothesized that individuals with a joint pathology adopt a gait reprogramming their movement patterns. Bhargava et al. found that following hip joint replacement patients' walking ability is reduced, even after successful hip replacement surgery. Studies of gait function show that although hip movements are pain-free in post replacement cases they are not normalized according to their age group. Symmetry of left to right foot parameters is not maintained because both hips do not equally share weight-bearing.

Dynamic loading is believed to play a significant role in the progression of knee OA. Morgenroth et al. found that the rate of dynamic loading at the knee was associated with increased medial tibiofemoral joint degenerative changes on MRI.

There have been numerous in vitro studies and in vivo animal studies suggesting the importance of the rate of loading in relation to the development of OA. Articular cartilage and underlying subchondral bone are viscoelastic structures that become less deformable when subjected to faster loading rates (Radin and Paul, 1971).

When articular cartilage is rapidly loaded, internal stresses can become quite large due to lack of fluid flow, and this can lead to fracture of the collagen matrix (Radin et al., 1991a). Subchondral bone can sustain microscopic damage with repetitive impulsive loads, which accumulate and can lead to subchondral stiffening (Radin et al., 1978, Radin and Rose, 1986), increasing shear stresses within articular cartilage thus leading to further degenerative changes (Anderson et al., 1993, Radin et al., 1991a).

Rapidly applied repetitive loading has been shown to cause joint damage as shown in vitro (Lukoschek et al., 1988) and in vivo animal models (Radin et al., 1984), even when load amplitude is within physiologic limits. For instance, when tested in rabbits in vivo, higher rate of loading led to cartilage degeneration more often than in animals with lower loading rate even though the latter had higher magnitudes of load (Yang, 1989).

The BVA Accepted this Author's IMO Regarding Osteoarthritis

DOCKET 15-33 431 11/22/2016

> "The Board finds that, affording the Veteran the benefit of the doubt, there is adequate probative medical evidence that his current low back disability is related to his in-service injury. Letters from private physician D.A. submitted in November 2015 and October 2016 discussed the Veteran's medical history, including the claimant's 1953 and 1956 back injuries. Although the physician did not have access to the Veteran's service treatment records, he did have what appears to be an accurate reporting of the claimant's in-service injuries. See *Nieves-Rodriguez v. Peake*, 22 Vet. App. 295, 303-304 (2008) (failure to review the claims file is not fatal to a medical opinion if the opinion is based on a correct factual premise). The physician also discussed medical literature regarding posttraumatic osteoarthritis, and he concluded that the Veteran's lumbar spine osteoarthritis was

more likely
than not due to his in-service injuries."

Understanding the Rating of Knee Injury

The Board most recently reviewed how rating of knee injuries should be performed [Citation Nr: 1302451 Decision Date: 01/23/13 Archive Date: 01/31/13 Docket No. 10-11 530] relating:

> "In determining the degree of limitation of motion, the provisions of 38 C.F.R. §§ 4.10, 4.40, and 4.45 are for consideration. *DeLuca v. Brown,* 8 Vet. App. 202 (1995)."

38 C.F.R. § 4.10 holds that the basis of disability evaluation is the ability of the body, system or organ of the body to function under the ordinary conditions of daily life including employment.

38 C.F.R. § 4.40 holds that disability of the musculoskeletal system is primarily the inability to perform the normal working movements of the body with normal excursion, strength, speed, coordination and endurance. Functional loss may be due to the absence or deformity of structures or other pathology, but it may also be due to pain, supported by adequate pathology and evidenced by the visible behavior in undertaking the motion. Weakness is as important as limitation of motion, and a part that becomes painful on use must be regarded as seriously disabled. With respect to joints, inquiry must be directed to weakened movement, excess fatigability, incoordination, pain on movement, swelling, deformity or atrophy of disuse.

38 C.F.R. § 4.45 holds that degenerative arthritis established by x-ray findings is evaluated under Diagnostic Code 5003, which in turn is evaluated based on the limitation of motion under the appropriate diagnostic code for the specific joint involved.

- **Knee Anatomy**

The knee is one of the largest and most complex joints in the body. The knee joins the thigh bone (femur) to the shin bone (tibia). The smaller bone that runs alongside the tibia (fibula) and the kneecap (patella) are the other bones that make the knee joint.

Tendons connect the knee bones to the leg muscles that move the knee joint. Ligaments join the knee bones and provide stability to the knee. The anterior cruciate ligament prevents the femur from sliding backward on the tibia (or the tibia sliding forward on the femur). The posterior cruciate ligament prevents the femur from sliding forward on the tibia (or the tibia from sliding backward on the femur). The medial and lateral collateral ligaments prevent the femur from sliding side to side.

Two C-shaped pieces of cartilage called the medial and lateral menisci act as shock absorbers between the femur and tibia. Numerous bursae, or fluid-filled sacs, help the knee move smoothly.

- **Knee Conditions**

Chondromalacia patella (also called patellofemoral syndrome): Irritation of the cartilage on the underside of the kneecap (patella), causing knee pain. This is a common cause of knee pain in young people.

Knee osteoarthritis: Osteoarthritis is the most common form of arthritis, and often affects the knees. Caused by aging and wear and tear of cartilage, osteoarthritis symptoms may include knee pain, stiffness, and swelling.

Knee effusion: Fluid buildup inside the knee, usually from inflammation. Any form of arthritis or injury may cause a knee effusion.

Meniscal tear: Damage to a meniscus, the cartilage that cushions the knee, often occurs with twisting the knee. Large tears may cause the knee to lock.

ACL (anterior cruciate ligament) strain or tear: The ACL is responsible for a large part of the knee's stability. An ACL tear often leads to the knee "giving out," and may require surgical repair.

PCL (posterior cruciate ligament) strain or tear: PCL tears can cause pain, swelling, and knee instability. These injuries are less common than ACL tears, and physical therapy (rather than surgery) is usually the best option.

MCL (medial collateral ligament) strain or tear: This injury may cause pain and possible instability to the inner side of the knee.

Patellar subluxation: The kneecap slides abnormally or dislocates along the thigh bone during activity. Knee pain around the kneecap results.

Patellar tendonitis: Inflammation of the tendon connecting the kneecap (patella) to the shin bone. This occurs mostly in athletes from repeated jumping.

Knee bursitis: Pain, swelling, and warmth in any of the bursae of the knee. Bursitis often occurs from overuse or injury.

Baker's cyst: Collection of fluid in the back of the knee. Baker's cysts usually develop from a persistent effusion as in conditions such as arthritis.

Rheumatoid arthritis: An autoimmune condition that can cause arthritis in any joint, including the knees. If untreated, rheumatoid arthritis can cause permanent joint damage.

Gout: A form of arthritis caused by buildup of uric acid crystals in a joint. The knees may be affected, causing episodes of severe pain and swelling.

Pseudo gout: A form of arthritis similar to gout, caused by calcium pyrophosphate crystals depositing in the knee or other joints.

Septic arthritis: Bacterial infection inside the knee can cause inflammation, pain, swelling, and difficulty moving the knee. Although uncommon, septic arthritis is a serious condition that usually gets worse quickly without treatment.

- **Limitation of Motion**

Knee injury is very common among servicemen. The injury may be slight, but years later, many veterans develop severe knee arthritis attributed to their initial service injury. Many veterans are so disabled by their knee arthritis that they are unable to work. Regrettably, the ratings for knee disability are outdated and have not been revised for many years. Thus, most knee disability claims are granted only a 10% to 20% disability rating. Veterans unable to maintain gainful employment due to their knee disability cannot apply for unemployability because their disabling condition is only rated at 20%.

One can clearly see by reviewing the rating tables below that the maximal rating for the common knee injuries is 30%.

5256 Knee, ankylosis of:	
Extremely unfavorable, in flexion at an angle of 45° or more	60
In flexion between 20° and 45°	50
In flexion between 10° and 20°	40
Favorable angle in full extension, or in slight flexion between 0° and 10°	30

Ankylosis means that the knee is fixed; flexion and extension of the knee is at best incomplete. The rating for knee ankylosis will not be addressed further here, as this condition is extremely rare due to advances in knee surgery.

5257 Knee, other impairment of:	
Recurrent subluxation or lateral instability:	
Severe	30
Moderate	20
Slight	10

Severe - Documented instability that is not correctable by bracing and that interferes with activities of daily living (30)

Moderate - Documented instability that is correctable by bracing, but that interferes at times with activities of daily living and prevents activities such as running and jumping (20)

Slight - Documented instability that is correctable by bracing and that does not interfere with activities of daily living, but at times may interfere with activities such as running and jumping (10)

(Note: Combine with an evaluation of pain (under § 4.59) when appropriate.)

5258 Cartilage, semilunar, dislocated, with frequent episodes of "locking," pain, and effusion into the joint	20
5259 Cartilage, semilunar, removal of, symptomatic	10
5260 Leg, limitation of flexion of:	
Flexion limited to 15°	30
Flexion limited to 30°	20
Flexion limited to 45°	10
Flexion limited to 60°	0
5261 Leg, limitation of extension of:	
Extension limited to 45°	50
Extension limited to 30°	40
Extension limited to 20°	30
Extension limited to 15°	20
Extension limited to 10°	10
Extension limited to 5°	0

5055 Knee replacement (prosthesis).	
Prosthetic replacement of knee joint:	
For 1 year following implantation of prosthesis	100
With chronic residuals consisting of severe painful motion or weakness in the affected extremity	60
With intermediate degrees of residual weakness, pain or limitation of motion rate by analogy to diagnostic codes 5256, 5261, or 5262.	
Minimum rating	30

In 2003, the VA, after extensive studies, provided an amendment to the rating for musculoskeletal injuries. This was published in the Federal Register Vol. 68, No. 28/Tuesday, February 11, 2003/Proposed Rules:

Knee replacement (diagnostic code 5055 Total or partial knee arthroplasty or replacement (with prosthesis):

From date of hospital admission for arthroplasty, either initial or revision (100)

Requiring use of two crutches or a walker for ambulation (90)

Requiring use of one crutch or two canes for most ambulation, due to pain, instability, or weakness (muscle strength grade zero to 2 out of 5); or with loss of more than 40 degrees of the full arc of motion (70)

Requiring use of one crutch or two canes only for ambulating long distances (500 feet or more), due to pain, instability, or weakness (muscle strength grade 3 to 4 out of 5); or with loss of 21 to 40 degrees of the full arc of motion (50)

Requiring use of one cane or brace for ambulation, due to pain, instability, or weakness; or with loss of 10 to 20 degrees of the full arc of motion (40)

Minimum evaluation following arthroplasty (30)

(Note (1): A full arc of motion of the knee after arthroplasty is a range of motion of 0 to 110 degrees.)

It is interesting to compare the rating of knee injuries to the rating of knee replacement. It is ironic, that after the veteran undergoes successful knee replacement resulting in reduced pain, stability and easier ambulation, the veteran is considered more disabled than he was before he underwent corrective surgery. The reason for this discrepancy is that the rating of knee replacement is rather new, while the rating for knee injury was created before World War II.

I argue that the same limitations used to rate knee replacement should also be used when rating knee injuries without knee replacement.

Evaluation of Pain

The Board also must consider a Veteran's pain, swelling, weakness, and excess fatigability when determining the appropriate rating for a disability using the limitation of motion diagnostic codes. 38 C.F.R. §§ 4.40, 4.45; see *DeLuca v. Brown*, 8 Vet. App. 202 (1995).

In *DeLuca*, the Court held:

> "The Board, however, based its evaluation of the disability entirely on the recorded limitation of motion. Although it is possible that the examiners considered the functional disability due to pain in determining the veteran's limitation of motion, neither the record nor the BVA decision contains clear indication that they did so. It seems no less plausible that the examiners may have recorded only the actual limitation of motion and may not have considered whether there was any additional disability due to pain or weakness of the left shoulder.
>
> Determination of whether the application of sections 4.40 and 4.45 entitles the veteran to an increased rating requires factual findings as to the extent to which the veteran's left-shoulder pain and weakness cause additional disability beyond that reflected in the measured limitation of his left-shoulder motion"

Additionally, VA General Counsel opinions provide for separate evaluations for knee instability and knee arthritis in certain cases. See 38 C.F.R. § 4.71a,

Diagnostic Codes 5003, 5010, 5260, 5261, 5257 (2012); see also VAOPGCPREC 23-97; 62 Fed. Reg. 63604 (1997) (knee arthritis and instability may be rated separately under Diagnostic Codes 5003 and 5257, provided that any separate rating is based upon additional disability); VAOPGCPREC 9-98; 63 Fed. Reg. 56704 (1998) (if a disability rating under Diagnostic Code 5257 for instability of the knee is in effect, and there is X-ray evidence of arthritis, a separate rating for arthritis based on painful motion can be assigned under 38 C.F.R. § 4.59).

In *Mitchell v. Shinseki* [No. 09-2169 8/2011] the United States Court of Appeals for Veteran Claims (CAVC) held that remand is warranted where the examiner did not reconcile a veteran's complaints of pain and fatigue with the examination that found minimal loss of movement on passive flexion and extension.

§ 4.59 Evaluation of pain in musculoskeletal conditions.

When the evaluation criteria for a condition in § 4.71a are based on signs and symptoms other than pain, and pain is a complaint, combine (do not add) the evaluation based on criteria other than pain with an evaluation for pain based on the following scale, and assign a single (combined) evaluation for the condition under the appropriate diagnostic code:

> (a) Complaint of pain that globally interferes with and severely limits daily activities; meets the requirement for a 30-% evaluation under this section; and a psychiatric evaluation has excluded other processes to account for the pain (100)

(b)   Complaint of pain at rest, with pain on minimal palpation or on attempted range of motion on physical examination; X-ray or other imaging abnormalities; and abnormal findings on a vascular or neurologic special study (30)

(c)   Complaint of pain on any use, with pain on palpation and through at least one-half of the range of motion on physical examination; and X-ray or other imaging abnormalities (20)

(d)   Complaint of pain on performing some daily activities, with pain on motion (through any part of the range of motion) on physical examination; and X-ray or other imaging abnormalities (10)

(e)   Complaint of mild or transient pain on performing some daily activities, with correlative finding(s) on physical examination (for example, pain on palpation or pain on stressing the joint), but without X-ray or other imaging abnormalities (0)

In 2003, the VA provided a handbook for the raters who perform the C&P evaluations. The handbook has been replaced by a computerized form, but it does indicate the importance the VA places on complying with CAVC holdings, specifically DeLuca.

How is the Functional Assessment of Joints Conducted?

Because the CAVC found that the traditional VA method of assessing disabilities for rating purposes – one-time measurement of active and passive ROM –

was inadequate under VA regulations, as functional impairment may be underestimated, additional factors must be considered for each joint examined. See *Deluca v. Brown*, 6 Vet. App. 321, 324 (1993). These include:

1) pain with joint movement
2) weakened movement against varying resistance
3) lack of endurance following repetitive use
4) effects of episodic exacerbations (flare-ups) on functional ability.

Each of these issues should be assessed and the amount the joint is additionally limited (if any) resulting from one or more of these factors should – if possible –be reported in degrees of additional loss of motion. The absence of any (or all) of these factors should also be noted. The evaluation must be specific as to where (i.e., from flexion or extension) any additional losses should be subtracted. For example, if knee pain on ROM testing prevents full flexion and an additional ROM loss for pain of 20 degrees is warranted, the examiner must specifically state the additional limitation of flexion due to pain (e.g., "An additional 20 degrees loss of knee flexion is warranted because of pain on movement" or, better and clearer, "Because of pain on movement, the ROM is estimated to be 0 to X rather than 0 to Y found on range of motion without taking pain into consideration."). At present, there are no guidelines as to which tests should be used to determine the strength and endurance for the various joints. These tests should be individualized, keeping in mind patient safety.

Example: If shoulder abduction is 0 to 180 degrees against gravity, but there is evidence of pain (verbal complaint, facial grimace, etc.) between 120 degrees and 180 degrees, this should be documented. If further testing for endurance against resistance (e.g., 10 repetitions using a 5-pound dumbbell) reduces shoulder abduction to 90 degrees, this should be reported. If more than one factor is contributing to loss of ROM, it should be stated – if possible – which has the major functional impact. This can be done as a comment. For the above example, this might read: "Comment: While shoulder abduction against gravity is full, 0 to 180 degrees, because of the combined effects of pain and lack of endurance, the veteran's functional ROM is best estimated to be 0 to 90 degrees."

The examiner should describe the patient's functional disability as to effects on daily activities (eating, dressing, walking, breathing, etc.) and employment.

Combined Rating and the Rule Against Pyramiding

The VA frequently will address only one disability rather than all the conditions raised by the veteran. For example, if the veteran has limitation of motion, knee instability as well as surgery for removal of the meniscus the VA will simply choose one of the three often arguing that the rule against pyramiding allows for such. The law provides that a veteran is entitled to a separate disability evaluation when an injury manifests in two different disabilities. Under 38 C.F.R. § 4.14 – "Avoidance of Pyramiding," the rule provides that evaluation of the same disability (or manifestation of disability) under various/different diagnoses is to be avoided. As long as the symptoms do not overlap or are duplicative, then the rule against pyramiding set forth in section 4.14 isn't violated.

Esteban v. Brown, 6 Vet. App. 259, 261-262 (1994) clarifies the application of this law. Veteran was injured on right side of face in motor vehicle accident in January 1949 in Okinawa. He sustained four scars (slight to moderate disfigurement), injury to facial muscles, and pain on right side of face. The BVA denied his claim for injury to his facial muscles and pain to his face and limited his benefits to the scars and assigned a 10% rating under DC 7800 for moderately disfiguring scars. The court rejected the BVA analysis. It held that the summary conditions could be rated separately unless they constitute the "same disability" or the "same manifestation" under 38 C.F.R. § 4.14. The support for establishing three separate disabilities is that "none of the symptomatology for any of the 3 conditions is duplicative of or overlapping with symptomatology of the other 2 conditions". Veteran's symptomatology is distinct and separate:

(1) disfigurement;
(2) painful scars; and
(3) facial damage resulting in problems with mastication (chewing)

Thus, the court concluded that, as a matter of law, Veteran is entitled to combine (under 38 C.F.R. § 4.25) his 10% rating for disfigurement under DC 7800 with an additional 10% rating for tender and painful scars under DC 7804 and a third 10% rating for facial muscle injury interfering with mastication under DC 5325.

Pursuant to the Esteban holding the Veterans' Administration General Counsel provided an opinion binding on the VA (VA Gen. Coun. Prec. Op. 23-97 (July 1,1997):

> "limitation of motion and instability may be rated separately under DCs 5003, 5260, or 5261 for limitation of motion and DC 5257 for instability. Pursuant to this decision, the disability listed in the following rating code can be combined:
>
> DC   5003 - Degenerative Arthritis
>
> DC   5260 - Limitation of Flexion
>
> DC   5261 - Limitation of Extension
>
> DC   5257 - Recurrent Subluxation or Lateral Instability
>
> Because none of the symptoms addressed in the limitation of motion DCs (DCs 5003, 5260, 5261) duplicate or otherwise overlap under another opinion (VA Gen. Coun. Prec. Op. 9-98), a separate rating for arthritis could also be based on X-ray findings and painful motion under 38 C.F.R. § 4.59, per *Lichtenfels v. Derwinski*, 1 Vet.App. 484 (1991). The Lichtenfels court held that the VA must combined, DC 5003, and §4.59 and thus painful motion of a major joint or groups caused by degenerative arthritis. Where the arthritis is established by X-ray is deemed to be limited motion and entitled to a minimum 10%

rating, per joint, even though there is no actual limitation of motion."

A more recent decision by the CAVC (*Burton v. Shinseki*, 25 Vet.App. 1 (2011) held that painful motion even without x-ray findings of arthritis may also warrant a separate compensable rating under 38 C.F.R. § 4.59. VA Gen. Coun. Prec. Op. 9-2004 (Sept.17, 2004) Separate ratings under DC 5260 (leg, limitation of flexion) and DC 5261 (leg, limitation of extension), may be assigned for disability of the same joint.

Proposed Amendment to the Rating of Musculoskeletal Conditions

After extensive studies, in 2003, the VA provided an amendment to the rating for musculoskeletal injuries which was published in the Federal Register /Vol. 68, No. 28/Tuesday, February 11, 2003/Proposed Rules. Mysteriously, despite any objection to the proposed rules, the new rating codes were not incorporated in the rating guidelines. I argue that these new rules are binding on the Veterans' Administration.

In *Gerard Cullen v. Eric K. Shinseki*, United States Court of Appeals for Veterans Claims 24 Vet. App. 74; 2010 U.S. App. Vet. Claims LEXIS 1477 No. 08-1193 June 10, 2010, Cullen argued that the VA did not adequately provide separate ratings for his lumbar spine injuries. The VA, realizing the weaknesses of the current rating codes, argued before the Court that they actually rely on the proposed amendment rule that was published 10 years earlier. The Court held that they must provide substantial deference to the proposed amendments offered by the VA:

> "Turning to VA's notice of proposed rulemaking, published in the Federal Register in September 2002 (prior to the final rule's enactment in November 2003... [T]he Court concludes that VA's position is consistent both with the regulation itself and with VA's demonstrated interpretation of the regulation and is therefore due substantial deference from the Court. *See Auer*, 519 U.S. at 461-62; *Cathedral Candle Co.*, 400 F.3d at 1364"

I assert that since the old ratings have not been replaced by the new ratings, an advocate should ask the BVA to accept their own proposed rule as binding.

The following excerpts of the publications can be found in Knee and Lower Leg Federal Register /Vol. 68, No. 28/Tuesday, February 11, 2003/ Proposed Rules:

> "Diagnostic code 5257 is currently titled ''Knee, other impairment of,'' but the criteria are based only on the extent of recurrent subluxation or lateral instability. Thirty % is assigned if the condition is ''severe,'' 20% if it is ''moderate,'' and 10% if it is ''slight.'' The proposed amendment, provides a 30% evaluation if there is documented instability that is not correctable by bracing and that interferes with activities of daily living; a 20% evaluation if there is documented instability that is correctable with bracing, but that interferes at times with activities of daily living and that prevents activities such as running and jumping; and a 10% evaluation if there is documented instability that is correctable by

bracing and that does not interfere with activities of daily living, but at times may interfere with activities such as running and jumping. The VA proposes to add a note directing that an evaluation under diagnostic code 5257 may be combined with an evaluation for pain (under § 4.59).

Diagnostic code 5258 is currently titled "Cartilage, semilunar, dislocated, with frequent episodes of 'locking,' pain, and effusion into the joint". It provides a single evaluation level of 20%. The VA proposes to provide a 20% evaluation for meniscus injury with episodes of giving way, locking, or joint effusion that interfere at times with activities of daily living and prevent activities such as running and jumping, and a 10% evaluation for meniscus injury with episodes of giving way, locking, or joint effusion that do not interfere with activities of daily living, but that at times interfere with activities such as running and jumping. The VA also proposes that evaluation alternatively be based on instability, degenerative arthritis, etc., depending on the specific findings, under the appropriate diagnostic code, because these are possible effects of meniscus injury or surgery. The VA also proposes to add a note directing that an evaluation under diagnostic code 5258 be combined with an evaluation for pain (under § 4.59) when appropriate.

Diagnostic codes 5260 and 5261 currently pertain to limitation of flexion of the leg and limitation of extension of the leg, respectively. Because the terms extension and flexion are functions of the knee joint, flexion of the knee limited to 15 degrees is currently evaluated at 30%, flexion limited to 30 degrees is evaluated at 20%, flexion limited to 45 degrees is evaluated at 10%, and flexion limited to 60 degrees is evaluated at 0%. Based on the VHA Orthopedic Committee the VA proposes to provide a 30-% evaluation if flexion is limited to 30 degrees, a 20- % evaluation if it is limited to 60 degrees, and a 10-% evaluation if it is limited to 90 degrees.

Under diagnostic code 5261, currently "Leg, limitation of extension," current evaluations are 50 % if extension is limited to 45 degrees, 40 % if it is limited to 30 degrees, 30 % if it is limited to 20 degrees, 20 % if it is limited to 15 degrees, 10 % if it is limited to 10 degrees, and zero % if it is limited to 5 degrees. The VA proposes to provide evaluation levels of 50 % if extension is limited to more than minus 30 degrees (lacks more than 30 degrees of full extension), 30 % if extension is limited to between minus 16 and 30 degrees (lacks 16 to 30 degrees of full extension), and 10 % if extension is limited to between minus 5 and 15 degrees (lacks 5 to 15 degrees of full extension)."

Understanding the New Rating Table for Cervical and Lumbar Spine Disability

Degenerative joint disease of the spine is one of the most common claims made by veterans for service-connected disability, since back injury is so common during military service. Contrast back injury with other conditions, such as cardiac conditions, which rarely affect young soldiers.

An injury to the spine can result in severe limitations, leaving a veteran unable to work. It is, thus, surprising that veterans are granted disability ratings of only 10% to 20% for back injuries, while higher ratings, and even Individual Unemployability, are granted for conditions like depression or cardiac disease. The reason for this discrepancy is the history of disability rating.

The rating table was created before World War I and was based on medical science existing at that time. The VA has been very resistant to updates and upgrades of its rating index. The VA has added new and modern rating classifications for mental disease and cardiac disease which conform with the newest accepted classifications by the American Medical Association, but progress in updating the ratings of common musculoskeletal ailments is slow. Recently, the VA did allow some modifications to its rating of degenerative joint disease of the back and neck. Knowledge of the subtleties involved in the rating of this condition is important for a successful and fair rating of a veteran's service-connected disability.

Central to understanding the old classification is the term "ankylosis," which describes a joint that does not move or is very limited in its motion. The VA requires that the examiner measure the maximal flexion and extension of the joints using a goniometer. The VA still uses this classification for most disabilities affecting the joints and for evaluation of degenerative joint disease of the spine. The VA uses ankylosis in providing ratings for the following conditions:

5235 Vertebral fracture or dislocation
5236 Sacroiliac injury and weakness
5237 Lumbosacral or cervical strain
5238 Spinal stenosis
5239 Spondylolisthesis or segmental instability
5240 Ankylosing spondylitis
5241 Spinal fusion
5242 Degenerative arthritis of the spine (see also diagnostic code 5003)

Unfavorable ankylosis is extremely rare in clinical practice. It means that the entire spine is in flexion; a person cannot move his spine at all.

> *Unfavorable ankylosis of the entire cervical spine; or, forward flexion of the thoracolumbar spine 30 degrees or less; or, favorable ankylosis of the entire thoracolumbar spine (40)*

> *Forward flexion of the cervical spine 15 degrees or less; or, favorable ankylosis of the entire cervical spine (30)*

Using the rating table for unfavorable ankylosis will result in a rating no higher than 40%. Note, that even if the veteran is totally unemployable, he cannot file for individual unemployability with a rating of only 40%.

What is Intervertebral Disc Syndrome (IVDS)?

IVDS is a group of signs and symptoms resulting from displacement of an intervertebral disc or disc fragments at any level of the spine. There are usually pain and other signs and symptoms at or near the site of the disc, and there may be pain referred to more remote areas, plus neurologic abnormalities due to irritation or pressure on adjacent nerves or nerve roots. IVDS may also be referred to as a slipped, herniated, or ruptured disc, degenerative disc disease (DDD) or sciatica. In the case of lumbar disc disease, IVDS commonly includes back pain and sciatica (pain along the course of the sciatic nerve into the buttock and the leg). In the case of cervical disk, IVDS will present with neck pain and radiating arm or hand pain.

Lumbar IVDS accounts for 62% of all disc disease. All but 10% of lumbar IVDS is at the L4-L5 or L5-S1 level. Cervical IVDS accounts for 36% of all disc disease. The C6-C7 level is the most common location of cervical IVDS, followed by the C5-C6 level. IVDS is uncommon in the thoracic area, where the spine is less mobile.
- **The pertinent anatomy for IVDS**

Two anatomic areas are of importance in IVDS: the spine itself and the area(s) innervated by any nerves that are affected due to compression of the nerve roots, spinal nerves, or spinal cord by a displaced disc or disc fragments.

Spine

The vertebral column is made up of 33 bony vertebrae: 7 cervical, 12 thoracic, 5 lumbar, 5 sacral (fused into one bone, the sacrum), and 4 coccygeal (fused into one bone, the coccyx). The vertebral bodies are separated from one another by intervertebral discs, which are spongy circular cushions made up of cartilage and fibrous tissue. Each disc consists of a tough outer ring called the annulus fibrosis and an inner softer, jelly-like, core called the nucleus pulposus. The upper and lower surfaces of a disc are the cartilaginous endplates.

Discs, or intervertebral discs, are named according to the number of the vertebrae above and below. Therefore, the disc between the second and third lumbar vertebrae is called the L2-L3 disc, and the disc between the fifth lumbar and first sacral vertebrae is called the L5-S1 disc.

Nerves

Each segment of the spinal cord gives off a ventral or anterior motor nerve root and a dorsal or posterior sensory nerve root. These two roots join to form a spinal nerve at each segment of the spine. The nerve roots themselves may be damaged by disc disease, but they are particularly vulnerable to pressure from disc disease at the point at which the two roots unite.

Irritation or compression of a nerve root by disc disease may lead to pain and other symptoms.

Nerve root damage from any cause is called radiculopathy. Radiculitis means inflammation of a nerve root and is sometimes used interchangeably with radiculopathy. Radicular refers to the nerve root (or radicle) of a nerve.

- **Cause of IVDS**

With aging, the disc tends to dry out and shrink, causing the annulus fibrosis to deteriorate and bulge outward. This is a bulging disc. With continued degeneration, due to mechanical stress, wear and tear, or trauma, the annulus may tear and allow the nucleus pulposus to extrude or rupture through the tear into the spinal canal. This is a ruptured or herniated disc.

- **Symptoms of IVDS**

Lumbar IVDS

Pain - Back pain may be the primary symptom, but pain in the distribution of the irritated or compressed nerve root may also be primary. However, some people have no back pain at all. There may also be referred pain in the buttocks, sacroiliac joints, and thighs. Referred pain is pain perceived in an area of the body that is far away from the site of pathology.

There may be sciatica, which is sharp, burning, or stabbing pain radiating from the low back down the posterior thigh and posterolateral lower leg, and possibly into the side of the foot. It is due to S1 or L5 radiculopathy.

Pain is worse when sitting and standing than when lying down. Coughing, sneezing, bending, or heavy lifting may aggravate the pain.

Sensory abnormality - The exact area of numbness or other abnormal sensations, if any, is determined by the particular nerve root affected, and may be in the inner ankle, the great toe, the heel, the outer ankle, the outer leg, or a combination.

Motor abnormality - Weakness or paralysis depends on the particular nerve root affected, and may affect ankle upward or downward motion or dorsiflexion of the great toe on the affected side.

Reflexes - There may be abnormal deep tendon reflexes of knee (patellar) or ankle (Achilles tendon).

Cervical IVDS

Pain - Neck pain

Pain radiating down the arm (brachialgia). The pain may be sharp, burning, stinging, or stabbing in the arm, elbow, wrist or fingers, depending on the disc site. It is the upper extremity equivalent of sciatica in the lower extremity. There may be referred pain in the upper middle of the back. Headache is common.

C5-C6 IVDS may include weakness of elbow flexion and wrist extension and sensory loss of lateral forearm, thumb, and lateral part of index finger.

C6-C7 IVDS may include pain in the lateral forearm, thumb, and index finger; weakness of elbow and wrist extension; sensory loss of the long finger; and a decreased triceps reflex.

- **Diagnosis of IVDS**

Clinical findings are always a significant factor in diagnosis because neurodiagnostic imaging studies show positive findings in at least one-third of patients who are free of symptoms.

X rays: Can demonstrate bony alignment and may show decreased disc height, but do not show a disc fragment compressing a nerve. Have limited value because degenerative changes are age-related and are equally present in asymptomatic and symptomatic persons. However, they help rule out tumors, infections, and fractures.

Magnetic Resonance Imaging (MRI): Is *the gold standard* for visualizing a herniated disc. It can show annular tears and other anatomic details. Does not require an injection.

Computed Tomography Myelogram (CT Myelogram): A myelogram is an x-ray taken after contrast material is injected into the spinal canal to outline the spinal cord and nerves. Herniated disc fragments or bone spurs compressing the nerves are well visualized, but it is inferior to MRI in soft tissue detail. Largely replaced by MRI, which does not require injection.

Electromyogram and Nerve Conduction Studies (EMG/NCS): Done in selected cases to assess function of a compressed nerve.

Discography: Injection of contrast material directly into a disc. Usually done with CT.

- **Treatment of IVDS**

Conservative therapy - The first line of treatment, unless there is severe nerve involvement, may include any or all of the following:

- limited bed rest (2-7 days generally, but rarely up to 2 to 4 weeks)
- physical therapy, such as ultrasound, heat or ice, massage, conditioning, and exercise programs
- traction
- electric nerve stimulation
- trigger point injections
- weight control
- lumbosacral back support - braces or corsets
- medications, such as analgesics, anti-inflammatory drugs, and muscle relaxants

Most patients recover within four weeks of onset of symptoms, regardless of type of treatment. Sciatica resolves in 75% of patients within six months. When conservative therapy fails (which occurs in about 10%), surgery may be needed.

Indications for surgery:

- progressive neurologic deficit
- profound neurologic deficit
- severe and disabling pain refractory to 4 to 6 weeks of conservative treatment
- cauda equina syndrome

Common types of surgery

- Laminectomy: traditional surgery performed for lumbar IVDS to relieve pressure on one or more nerve roots. The posterior arch of the spine (lamina) is removed to create more space for the nerve root, in order to relieve compression. Part of the disc may be removed, as may bony spurs and scar tissue.

- Laminotomy: newer, less invasive type of surgery for lumbar IVDS, in which only the small area of the lamina directly surrounding the affected disk, instead of the whole back of the lamina, is removed. This keeps the spine more stable.

- Anterior cervical decompression, with or without fusion: surgery for cervical IVDS, in which the disc material is removed and the spine may be fused at the level of the abnormal disc.

After successful surgery, 80-85% of patients do extremely well and are able to return to work in about six weeks. Small areas of leg numbness may remain. Mild flare-ups of sciatic type pain occasionally develop.

- **Rating for IVDS**

IVDS can be rated in two ways. One is to look for the extent of incapacitating episodes. The other is to look for objective signs and symptoms of IVDS, specifically nerve or orthopedic damage. The Veterans' Administration will allow a veteran only the highest rating of the two and does not allow combining of the two to get a higher rating.

IVDS that is primarily disabling because of periods of acute symptoms that require bedrest according to the cumulative amount of time over the course of a year that the patient is incapacitated, i.e., requires bedrest and treatment by a physician, is evaluated:

- 60% if there are incapacitating episodes of at least six weeks' total duration during the past 12 months;
- 40% if there are incapacitating episodes of at least four but less than six weeks' total duration during the past 12 months;

- 20% if there are incapacitating episodes of at least two but less than four weeks' total duration during the past 12 months;
- 10% if there are incapacitating episodes of at least one but less than two weeks' total duration during the past 12 months.

IVDS that is disabling primarily because of chronic orthopedic manifestations (e.g., painful muscle spasm or limitation of motion), chronic neurologic manifestations (e.g., foot drop, muscle weakness or atrophy, or sensory loss), or a combination of both, is evaluated by assigning separate evaluations for the orthopedic and neurologic manifestations, using diagnostic code 5293 hyphenated with the appropriate orthopedic (musculoskeletal) or neurologic code.

When IVDS is disabling both because of incapacitating episodes and persistent orthopedic or neurologic manifestations, whichever alternative method of evaluation results in a higher evaluation is used.

The great majority of cases will be more favorably evaluated under the second method.

To determine which method results in the higher evaluation:

1) Calculate the percentage evaluation based on the cumulative amount of time over the course of the past 12 months that the patient is incapacitated,

and combine with the evaluation for all other service-connected disabilities.
2) Calculate the percentage evaluation based on the orthopedic and neurologic manifestations, and combine with the evaluation for all other service-connected disabilities.
3) Compare the two overall evaluations, and assign an evaluation for IVDS based on the method that results in the higher evaluation.

- **Incapacitating Episodes**

The regulation requires for incapacitating episodes that there be periods of acute symptoms that require bed rest. However, the treatment of back pain by bed rest has been now abandoned. The American College of Physicians and the American Pain Society provided the following guidelines for the treatment of back pain (excerpts are from Diagnosis and Treatment of Low Back Pain: A Joint Clinical Practice Guideline from the American College of Physicians and the American Pain Society Ann Intern Med. 2007;147:478-491):

> "General advice on self-management for nonspecific low back pain should include recommendations to remain active, which is more effective than resting in bed for patients with acute or subacute low back pain (65, 66). If patients require periods of bed rest to relieve severe symptoms, they should be encouraged to return to normal activities as soon as possible."

Instead of bed rest, the panel recommended:

"Recommendation 7: For patients who do not improve with selfcare options, clinicians should consider the addition of nonpharmacologic therapy with proven benefits — for acute low back pain, spinal manipulation; for chronic or subacute low back pain, intensive interdisciplinary rehabilitation, exercise therapy, acupuncture, massage therapy, spinal manipulation, yoga, cognitive-behavioral therapy, or progressive relaxation (weak recommendation, moderate-quality evidence)."

It appears that even the Veterans' Administration has accepted this recommendation. In a training letter to its staff, the VA stated (emphasis added):

"How is IVDS treated?
Conservative therapy - the first line of treatment unless there is severe nerve involvement. May include any or all of the following:
limited bed rest (2-7 days generally, but rarely up to 2 to 4 weeks)
physical therapy, such as ultrasound, heat or ice, massage, conditioning, and exercise programs
traction
electric nerve stimulation
trigger point injections
weight control
lumbosacral back support - braces or corsets
medications, such as analgesics, anti-inflammatory drugs, and muscle relaxants"

It is recommended, therefore, that in a case when a veteran's back pain was so severe that it required physical therapy, enhanced drugs including narcotics, and multiple visits to physicians and healthcare providers, that the veteran's advocate argue that the time expended in using these modalities should be equivalent to "bed rest" used in the regulation to prove incapacitation. At this point, neither the BVA nor the Courts have reviewed such arguments, but I believe that pressure from veterans and advocates taking this approach will eventually result in acceptance. Meanwhile a veteran is instructed to report bed rest to his physician and to keep a diary as evidence. Calculation of bed rest is cumulative; a veteran does not need continuous 6 weeks of bed rest.

What Does a VA Examiner Look for in Musculoskeletal Rating?

During the claim process a veteran will undoubtedly be required to undergo an evaluation by a Veterans' Administration examiner. However, it is recommended that the veteran also ask his treating physician to provide a detailed clinical examination with pertinent findings, which will allow the advocate to claim that the examination by the VA personnel was inadequate.

Straight leg raising (SLR) is a test is done by gently lifting the relaxed, extended lower extremity to approximately 90 degrees, with the patient lying supine. This stretches the sciatic nerve and reproduces sciatic pain. The normal limit without pain when there is no sciatic nerve abnormality is between 60 and 120 degrees, depending on the patient's age, habitus, and physical condition. The amount of pain-free flexion is less important than variation between the legs. SLR, while sensitive, is non-specific because it may be limited or painful due to tight hamstring muscles, sacro-iliac joint pathology, or radiculitis.

Lasegues sign is worsening of the pain in an SLR test by dorsiflexing the foot. The hallmark is pain. This may be associated with abnormal sensations (paresthesias) such as tingling or increased sensitivity, or with sensory loss in a dermatomal distribution. There may be weakness of muscles innervated by the nerve root.

Signs Suggesting that a Veteran is Malingering or Exaggerating His Symptoms

The VA examiner will look for evidence that a veteran is exaggerating his symptoms or is simply a malingerer. A veteran must be careful not to exaggerate his symptoms. Waddell's signs may be interpreted as exaggeration of symptoms designed to get a higher rating, than actual anatomical injury.

These signs include:

- Superficial (skin) tenderness on light palpation. Positive when the skin is tender to light touch.
- Nonanatomic pain or tenderness. Positive when there is pain or tenderness extending over a wider area than that expected from the nerve pinched.

- Axial loading that increases pain. Positive if pressing down on the top of the head of a standing patient produces low back pain. Positive if passive rotation of shoulders and pelvis to 30 degrees in a standing position causes back pain.
- Distracted straight-leg raise. Patient may complain of pain or limitation of motion in a normal SLR test, but not when examiner extends the knee with the patient seated, while examining the foot, etc. Such inconsistency is a positive sign.
- Regional sensory change. Positive if does not correspond to a neuroanatomic or dermatomal distribution, e.g., stocking or global distribution of numbness.
- Regional weakness. With true muscle weakness, there should be a smooth, non-jerky motion when range of motion is resisted. Positive if there is a sudden letting go of the muscle with cogwheeling, give-way, or breakaway weakness.
- Overreaction. Positive if there is inconsistent hypersensitivity to light touch or an exaggerated, nonreproducible response, such as excessive grimacing, tremors, etc. But cultural and individual differences, as well as observer bias, must be taken into consideration.
- McBride's test: Patient stands on one leg while raising the opposite knee to the chest. Because the knee is bent, no sciatic stretch occurs, and the spine is flexed, which removes pressure, so this should lessen low back pain. A reported increase

in pain, or a refusal to do the test, is a positive sign.
- Burns test: Patient is asked to kneel on a chair and touch the floor. Since the knees are bent, patients with true back pain or sciatica should be able to do the test without much difficulty. Those with nonorganic back pain usually cannot.

Degenerative Joint Disease Rating Based on Objective Tests

If the degenerative joint disease of the spine resulted in orthopedic or neurological damage, and if the rating for neurological damage exceeds the rating one can get for proving incapacitation, the advocate should look at the rating of nerve damage to the sciatic or peroneal nerve.

- **Sciatic Nerve Function**

The sciatic nerve is made up of nerve roots L4, L5, S1, S2, and S3. It supplies the muscles of the back of the knee and lower leg and sensation to the back of the thigh, part of the lower leg, and the sole of the foot. Incomplete damage may appear identical to damage to one of its branches (tibial or common peroneal nerve). Sensory abnormalities may include sensory changes of the back of the calf or the sole of the foot, such as numbness, tingling, burning, pins and needles sensation, other abnormal sensations, and any level of pain up to excruciating pain. Motor loss may include weakness of the knee or foot leading to difficulty walking, weakness or loss of knee flexion, and weakness or loss of foot inversion and plantar flexion. Reflexes may be abnormal, with weak or absent ankle-jerk reflex.

Sciatic nerve	
8520 Paralysis of:	
Complete; the foot dangles and drops, no active movement possible of muscles below the knee, flexion of knee weakened or (very rarely) lost	80
Incomplete:	
Severe, with marked muscular atrophy	60
Moderately severe	40

- **Common Peroneal Nerve Function**

The common peroneal nerve is derived from nerve roots L4, L5, S1, and S2. Sensory abnormalities may be loss of sensation, numbness, or tingling of the anterolateral lower leg and dorsum of foot & toes. Motor loss may include weakness or loss of dorsiflexion and eversion of foot, loss of extension of toes, and possibly footdrop. When selecting which code to use in a particular case of lumbar IVDS, note that common peroneal nerve function is limited to the lower leg and foot, while the sciatic nerve can affect the knee and even higher areas of the leg. Remember that sensory loss only should be rated at the mild, or at most, the moderate degree of peripheral nerve paralysis (See 38 CFR 4.124a in the paragraph introducing Diseases of the Peripheral Nerves.)

Anterior tibial nerve (deep peroneal)	
8523 Paralysis of:	
Complete; dorsal flexion of foot lost	30
Incomplete:	
Severe	20
Moderate	10

How do the New Evaluation Criteria for IVDS Compare to the Old Criteria?

The former evaluation criteria for IVDS (DC 5293) included:

- 60% evaluation for persistent sciatic neuropathy or other neurologic findings, with little intermittent relief;
- 40% evaluation for severe recurring attacks;
- 20% evaluation for moderate recurring attacks;
- 10% evaluation for a mild condition;
- 0% evaluation for the postoperative, cured condition.

These criteria required a subjective determination as to whether the condition is mild, moderate, or severe and raised questions as to when a 60% evaluation was warranted on the basis of neurologic manifestations. There was also uncertainty about whether IVDS with neurologic manifestations could be evaluated higher or lower than 60%. This subjectivity has been removed.

Alternative criteria allow evaluation under the method most beneficial to the veteran, and the revised criteria can all be applied to either the pre-operative or post-operative state.

- **Over evaluations**

Some raters have over evaluated IVDS by assigning 60% under diagnostic code 5293, and a separate 40% or 60% for sciatic or common peroneal nerve dysfunction, based in part on the same signs and symptoms. This represents pyramiding (per 4.14), since some of the same signs and symptoms (leg or foot weakness or sensory loss) were used to support two separate evaluations. *The revised evaluation criteria, where the (orthopedic) neck or back problems and the (neurologic) sensory or motor abnormalities remote from the disc site are evaluated separately, should eliminate this problem.*

Neuropathy

In the Schedule, diagnostic codes 5285-5295 apply to disabilities of the spine. 38 C.F.R. § 4.71a, DC 5285-5295 (1993). In evaluating a claim based on IVDS, the Schedule provides the following guidelines:

- Pronounced; with persistent symptoms, compatible with sciatic neuropathy with characteristic pain and demonstrable muscle spasm, absent ankle jerk, or other neurological findings appropriate to site of diseased disc, little intermittent relief (60)
- Severe; recurring attacks, with intermittent relief (40)
- Moderate; recurring attacks (20)
- Mild (10)
- Postoperative, cured (0)

38 C.F.R. § 4.71a, DC 5293 (1993).

Disabilities of the peripheral nerves are rated under a section of the Schedule entitled, "Neurological Conditions and Convulsive Disorders." 38 C.F.R. §§ 4.120-4.124a (1993). For a claim based upon paralysis of the external popliteal nerve (common peroneal), the Schedule provides:

External popliteal nerve (common peroneal)	
8521 Paralysis of:	
Complete; foot drop and slight drop of first phalanges of all toes, cannot dorsiflex the foot, extension (dorsal flexion) of proximal phalanges of toes lost; abduction of foot lost, adduction weakened; anesthesia covers entire dorsum of foot and toes	40
Incomplete:	
Severe	30
Moderate	20
Mild	10

Sciatic nerve	
8520 Paralysis of:	
Complete; the foot dangles and drops, no active movement possible of muscles below the knee, flexion of knee weakened or (very rarely) lost	80

Incomplete:	
Severe, with marked muscular atrophy	60
Moderately severe	40

The Board has determined (Citation Nr: 1334084 Decision Date: 10/28/13 Archive Date: 11/06/13):

> "The Veteran's service-connected peripheral neuropathy of the left and right lower extremities have been rated by the RO under the provisions of Diagnostic Code 8521 for paralysis of external popliteal nerve (common peroneal)."

The Board in Citation Nr: 1550087 Decision Date: 11/30/15 Archive Date: 12/04/15 held:

> "Neuritis, characterized by loss of reflexes, muscle atrophy, sensory disturbances, and constant pain, at times excruciating, is to be rated on the scale provided for injury of the nerve involved, with a maximum equal to severe incomplete paralysis. 38 C.F.R. § 4.123. Thus, neuritis, depending on its severity, can be assigned a 20% rating as listed for moderate incomplete paralysis or a 30% rating based on severe incomplete paralysis. 38 C.F.R. § 4.124a, Diagnostic Code 8622. Neuralgia, characterized usually by a dull and intermittent pain, of typical distribution so as to identify the nerve, is to be

rated on the same scale, with a maximum equal to moderate incomplete paralysis. 38 C.F.R. § 4.124. Thus, neuralgia can be assigned a maximum disability rating of 20%. 38 C.F.R. § 4.124a, Diagnostic Code 8722."

Ankle injury in paratroopers - Tarsal Tunnel Syndrome

Tarsal tunnel syndrome is a painful condition of the foot caused by pressure on the posterior tibial nerve as it passes along a passage called the tarsal tunnel just below the malleolus on the inside of the ankle. The condition is caused by over pronation.

In *Paratrooper's Ankle Fracture: Posterior Malleolar Fracture*, by Dr. Ki Won Young et al., fifty-six members of the special force brigade of the military who had sustained ankle fractures during parachute landings between January 2005 and April 2010 were retrospectively analyzed. There were 28 right and 28 left ankle fractures. Twenty-two patients had simple fractures and 34 patients had comminuted fractures. The average number of injury and fractures sites per person was 2.07 (116 injuries including a syndesmosis injury and a deltoid injury) and 1.75 (98 fracture sites), respectively. Twenty-three cases (41.07%) were accompanied by posterior malleolar fractures. Of the paratrooper ankle fractures, 41.07% were accompanied by posterior malleolar fractures, thus, paratrooper ankle fractures usually resulted in operative treatment. The most common injury mechanism was an external rotation injury that was rated by 55.36%. The ankle brace should be an important prevention method of ankle fractures. Supination-external rotation injuries were found in 20 cases, supination-adduction injuries in 22 cases, pronation-external rotation injuries in 11 cases, tibiofibular fractures in 2 cases, and simple medial malleolar fractures in 2 cases.

It is more likely than not that tarsal tunnel syndrome in a paratrooper is a result of multiple over pronation injuries during jumps in service. The condition should be rated as incomplete paralysis of the posterior tibial nerve; 10% for each lower extremity.

In another study, *Injuries in military parachuting: a prospective study of 4499 jumps*, Dr. A. Ekeland reported:

> "parachuting injuries which occurred during 2031 jumps in basic courses of free fall were compared with the injuries occurring during 2468 jumps for reserve paratroopers on training exercises. Fifty-eight injuries were recorded in 51 paratroopers. The ankle was most commonly affected, and 80% of the injuries involved the lower extremity."

5270 Ankle, ankylosis of:	
In plantar flexion at more than 40°, or in dorsiflexion at more than 10° or with abduction, adduction, inversion or eversion deformity	40
In plantar flexion, between 30° and 40°, or in dorsiflexion, between 0° and 10°	30
In plantar flexion, less than 30°	20

Rating for Shoulder Disability

5201 Arm, limitation of motion of:		
To 25° from side	40	30
Midway between side and shoulder level	30	20
At shoulder level	20	20

5202 Recurrent dislocation of at scapulohumeral joint.		
With frequent episodes and guarding of all arm movements	30	20
With infrequent episodes, and guarding of movement only at shoulder level	20	20
5203 Clavicle or scapula, impairment of:		
Dislocation of	20	20

5301 Group I. *Function:* Upward rotation of scapula; elevation of arm above shoulder level. *Extrinsic muscles of shoulder girdle:* (1) Trapezius; (2) levator scapulae; (3) serratus magnus	
Severe	40
Moderately Severe	30
Moderate	10
Slight	0
5302 Group II. *Function:* Depression of arm from vertical overhead to hanging at side (1, 2); downward rotation of scapula (3, 4); 1 and 2 act with Group III in forward and backward swing of arm. *Extrinsic muscles of shoulder girdle: (1) Pectoralis major II (costosternal); (2) latissimus dorsi and teres major (teres major, although technically an intrinsic muscle, is included with latissimus dorsi); (3) pectoralis minor; (4) rhomboid*	
Severe	40
Moderately Severe	30
Moderate	20
Slight	0
5303 Group III. *Function:* Elevation and abduction of arm to level of shoulder; act with 1 and 2 of Group II in forward and backward swing of arm. *Intrinsic muscles of*	

shoulder girdle: (1) Pectoralis major I (clavicular); (2) deltoid	
Severe	40
Moderately Severe	30
Moderate	20
Slight	0
5304 Group IV. *Function:* Stabilization of shoulder against injury in strong movements, holding head of humerus in socket; abduction; outward rotation and inward rotation of arm. *Intrinsic muscles of shoulder girdle: (1) Supraspinatus; (2) infraspinatus and teres minor; (3) subscapularis; (4) coracobrachialis*	
Severe	30
Moderately Severe	20
Moderate	10
Slight	0

CHAPTER 6 - CARDIOLOGY

Atherosclerosis and Coronary Risk Factors

Excerpts from Seshadri, S; R S, Vasan. Textbook of Medicine:

> "Atherosclerosis is the condition in which the inner layers of the arterial walls become thick and irregular because of fatty deposits mainly of cholesterol.
>
> Atherosclerotic lesions are commonly classified as one of three types: fatty streaks, fibrous plaques, and complicated lesions.
>
> The earliest lesions of atherosclerosis are the fatty streaks. The fatty streaks are universal in all children and begin in the aorta as early as in infancy. The fatty streaks contain about 25% lipid and are usually sessile and non-obstructive. A relationship between fatty streaks and subsequent fibrous plaques is presumptive. Fatty streaks are also found in the coronary arteries, usually in the third and fourth decade. The fibrous plaques consist of raised lesions of the arterial intima and represent the most characteristic lesion of atherosclerosis.
>
> Unlike the fatty streaks which are ubiquitous, fibrous plaques occur in subjects with advanced atherosclerosis. The fibrous plaques consist of a central core of extracellular lipid covered by a

fibromuscular cap of smooth muscle cells, macrophages, and collagen. The complicated lesion of atherosclerosis represents a calcified fibrous plaque with superimposed necrosis, ulceration and/ or thrombosis. The complicated lesions are frequently associated with acute symptoms."

Elevated Cholesterol Levels During Service Leads to Coronary Artery Disease

A report in the June 2008 issue of the American Journal of Roentgenology (AJR) highlighted the critical importance of quantifying plaque because the "total plaque burden is considered the most important predictor of coronary events." Furthermore, the article stated, "the rupture of soft noncalcified plaque has been implicated as the cause of heart attack."

The significance of plaque accumulation caused by the untreated hypercholesteremia and its progression was identified in a more recent series of randomized clinical arteriographic trials. The study showed that cholesterol plaques in all patients with control of their cholesterol would undergo abrupt progression to severe lesions by fissuring of atherosclerotic plaques. Clin. Cardiol. 17, 519-527 (1994), Brown BG. Bolson EL, Dodge HT: *Quantitative computer techniques for analyzing coronary arteriograms.* Progress in Cardiovascular Diseases 28, 403-418(1986) and Brown BG, Zhao X Q, Sacco DE, Alberts JJ: *Lipid lowering and plaque regression, new insights into prevention of plaque*

disruption and clinical events in coronary disease.
Circulation 87 1781-1791 (1993)

Particularly important for this discussion, is the Veterans' Administration's study on prevention of coronary artery disease by lowering cholesterol. The European Heart Journal addressed the VA HDL Intervention Trial: clinical implications, by Rubins HB, Robins SJ, Iwane MK et al.,*Rationale and design of the Department of Veterans Affairs High-Density Lipoprotein Cholesterol Intervention Trial (HIT) for secondary prevention of coronary artery disease in men with low high-density lipoprotein cholesterol and desirable low density lipoprotein cholesterol.* Am J Cardiol 1993; 71:45-52.

Rating of Coronary Artery Disease

The rating of coronary artery disease does not require full-fledged cardiac disability. It merely provides for "workload of greater than 3 METs but not greater than 5 METs resulting in dyspnea, fatigue, angina, dizziness, or syncope.

7005 Arteriosclerotic heart disease (Coronary artery disease):	
With documented coronary artery disease resulting in:	
Chronic congestive heart failure, or; workload of 3 METs or less results in dyspnea, fatigue, angina, dizziness, or syncope, or; left ventricular dysfunction with an ejection fraction of less than 30%	100
More than one episode of acute congestive heart failure in the past year, or; workload of greater than 3 METs but not greater than 5 METs results in dyspnea, fatigue, angina, dizziness, or syncope, or; left ventricular dysfunction with an ejection fraction of 30 to 50%	60
Workload of greater than 5 METs but not greater than 7 METs results in dyspnea, fatigue, angina, dizziness, or syncope, or; evidence of cardiac hypertrophy or dilatation on electrocardiogram, echocardiogram, or X-ray	30
Workload of greater than 7 METs but not greater than 10 METs results in dyspnea, fatigue, angina, dizziness, or syncope, or; continuous medication required	10

The Value of Stress Testing

In a recent case, a rating agency examiner stated that the veteran did not suffer from coronary artery disease because the stress tests performed were negative. An article entitled *Stress testing and non-invasive coronary angiography in patients with suspected coronary artery disease: time for a new paradigm*, by Dr. Armin Arbab-Zadeh, of the Division of Cardiology, Johns Hopkins University, shows that almost 18% suffer myocardial infarction or cardiac death after a normal pharmacological nuclear stress test. Thus, when assessing prognosis for patients based on stress testing results, it is important to consider the patient's co-morbidity and risk categorization. A normal stress test in a patient with significant co-morbidity by no means indicates a benign prognosis. An important limitation of stress testing is its inability to detect non-obstructive coronary atherosclerotic plaque, which is capable of triggering events.

Stress Testing and METS

Meaning of METS: One MET is the energy cost of standing quietly at rest and represents an oxygen uptake of 3.5 milliliters per kilogram of body weight per minute. This is the resting energy requirement. With progressive activity, the number of METs required progressively increases. For example, a workload of three METs represents such activities as level walking, driving, and very light calisthenics, and a workload of between three and five METs represents such activities as walking two and a half miles per hour, social dancing, light carpentry, etc.

ISCHEMIC HEART DISEASE (IHD) DISABILITY BENEFITS QUESTIONNAIRE OMB Approved No. 2900-0749:

This METs Level has been found to be consistent with activities such as:
☐ 1-3 METs (This METs level has been found to be consistent with activities such as eating, dressing, taking a shower, slow walking (2 mph) for 1-2 blocks)
☐ >3-5 METs (This METs /eve/ has been found to be consistent with activities such as light yard work (weeding), mowing lawn (power mower), brisk walking (4 mph)
☐ >5-7 METs (This METs le\el has been found to be consistent with activities such as golfing (without cart), mowing lawn (push mower), heavy yard work (digging)
☐ >7-10 METs (This METs level has been found to be consistent with activities such climbing stairs quickly. moderate bicycling, sawing

Daily activities with METS 0-5

05010 3.3 home activities cleaning, sweeping carpet or floors, general

05011 2.3 home activities cleaning, sweeping, slow, light effort

05012 3.8 home activities cleaning, sweeping, slow, moderate effort

05020 3.5 home activities cleaning, heavy or major (e.g. wash car, wash windows, clean garage), moderate effort

05021 3.5 home activities cleaning, mopping, standing, moderate effort

05022 3.2 home activities cleaning windows, washing windows, general

05023 2.5 home activities mopping, standing, light effort

05024 4.5 home activities polishing floors, standing, walking slowly, using electric polishing machine

05025 2.8 home activities multiple household tasks all at once, light effort

05026 3.5 home activities multiple household tasks all at once, moderate effort

05027 4.3 home activities multiple household tasks all at once, vigorous effort

05030 3.3 home activities cleaning, house or cabin, general, moderate effort

05032 2.3 home activities dusting or polishing furniture, general

05035 3.3 home activities kitchen activity, general, (e.g., cooking, washing dishes, cleaning up), moderate effort

05040 2.5 home activities cleaning, general (straightening up, changing linen, carrying out trash, light effort

05041 1.8 home activities wash dishes, standing or in general (not broken into stand/walk components)

05042 2.5 home activities wash dishes, clearing dishes from table, walking, light effort

05043 3.3 home activities vacuuming, general, moderate effort

05044 3.0 home activities butchering animals, small

05046 2.3 home activities cutting and smoking fish, drying fish or meat

05048 4.0 home activities tanning hides, general

05049 3.5 home activities cooking or food preparation, moderate effort

05050 2.0 home activities cooking or food preparation - standing or sitting or in general (not broken into stand/walk components), manual appliances, light effort

05051 2.5 home activities serving food, setting table, implied walking or standing

05052 2.5 home activities cooking or food preparation, walking

05053 2.5 home activities feeding household animals

05055 2.5 home activities putting away groceries (e.g. carrying groceries, shopping without a grocery cart), carrying packages

05057 3.0 home activities cooking Indian bread on an outside stove

05060 2.3 home activities food shopping with or without a grocery cart, standing or walking

05065 *2.3* home activities non-food shopping, with or without a cart, standing or walking

05070 1.8 home activities ironing

05080 1.3 home activities knitting, sewing, light effort, wrapping presents, sitting

05082 2.8 home activities sewing with a machine

05090 2.0 home activities laundry, fold or hang clothes, put clothes in washer or dryer, packing suitcase, washing clothes by hand, implied standing, light effort

05092 4.0 home activities laundry, hanging wash, washing clothes by hand, moderate effort

05095 2.3 home activities laundry, putting away clothes, gathering clothes to pack, putting away laundry, implied walking

05100 3.3 home activities making bed, changing linens

05110 5.0 home activities maple syruping/sugar bushing (including carrying buckets, carrying wood)

05121 5.0 home activities moving, lifting light loads

05125 4.8 home activities organizing room

05130 3.5 home activities scrubbing floors, on hands and knees, scrubbing bathroom, bathtub, moderate effort

05131 2.0 home activities scrubbing floors, on hands and knees, scrubbing bathroom, bathtub, light effort

05132 6.5 home activities scrubbing floors, on hands and knees, scrubbing bathroom, bathtub, vigorous effort

05140 4.0 home activities sweeping garage, sidewalk or outside of house

05146 3.5 home activities standing, packing or unpacking boxes, occasional lifting of lightweight household items, loading or unloading items in car, moderate effort

05147 3.0 home activities implied walking, putting away household items, moderate effort

05148 2.5 home activities watering plants

05149 2.5 home activities building a fire inside

05160 2.0 home activities standing, light effort tasks (pump gas, change light bulb, etc.)

05165 3.5 home activities walking, moderate effort tasks, non-cleaning (readying to leave, shut/lock doors, close windows, etc.)

05170 2.2 home activities sitting, playing with child(ren), light effort, only active periods

05171 2.8 home activities standing, playing with child(ren) light effort, only active periods

05175 3.5 home activities walking/running, playing with child(ren), moderate effort, only active periods

05181 3.0 home activities walking and carrying small child, child weighing 15 lbs or more

05182 2.3 home activities walking and carrying small child, child weighing less than 15 lbs.

05183 2.0 home activities standing, holding child

05184 2.5 home activities childcare, infant, general

05185 2.0 home activities child care, sitting/kneeling (e.g., dressing, bathing, grooming, feeding, occasional lifting of child), light effort, general

05186 3.0 home activities child care, standing (e.g., dressing, bathing, grooming, feeding, occasional lifting of child), moderate effort

05188 1.5 home activities reclining with baby

05189 2.0 home activities breastfeeding, sitting or reclining

05190 2.5 home activities sit, playing with animals, light effort, only active periods

05191 2.8 home activities stand, playing with animals, light effort, only active periods

05192 3.0 home activities walk/run, playing with animals, general, light effort, only active periods

05193 4.0 home activities walk/run, playing with animals, moderate effort, only active periods

05194 5.0 home activities walk/run, playing with animals, vigorous effort, only active periods

05195 3.5 home activities standing, bathing dog

05197 2.3 home activities animal care, household animals, general

05200 4.0 home activities elder care, disabled adult, bathing, dressing, moving into and out of bed, only active periods

05205 2.3 home activities elder care, disabled adult, feeding, combing hair, light effort, only active periods

06010 3.0 home repair airplane repair

06020 4.0 home repair automobile body work

06030 3.3 home repair automobile repair, light or moderate effort

06040 3.0 home repair carpentry, general, workshop (Taylor Code 620)

06050 6.0 home repair carpentry, outside house, installing rain gutters (Taylor Code 640), carpentry, outside house, building a fence

06052 3.8 home repair carpentry, outside house, building a fence

06060 3.3 home repair carpentry, finishing or refinishing cabinets or furniture

06070 6.0 home repair carpentry, sawing hardwood

06072 4.0 home repair carpentry, home remodeling tasks, moderate effort

06074 2.3 home repair carpentry, home remodeling tasks, light effort

06080 5.0 home repair caulking, chinking log cabin

06090 4.5 home repair caulking, except log cabin

06100 5.0 home repair cleaning gutters

06110 5.0 home repair excavating garage

06120 5.0 home repair hanging storm windows

06122 5.0 home repair hanging sheet rock inside house

06124 3.0 home repair hammering nails

06126 2.5 home repair, general, light effort

06127 4.5 home repair home repair, general, moderate effort

06130 4.5 home repair laying or removing carpet

06140 3.8 home repair laying tile or linoleum, repairing appliances

06144 3.0 home repair repairing appliances

06150 5.0 home repair painting, outside home (Taylor Code 650)

06160 3.3 home repair painting inside house, wallpapering, scraping paint

06165 4.5 home repair painting, (Taylor Code 630)

06167 3.0 home repair plumbing, general

06170 3.0 home repair put on and removal of tarp – sailboat

06190 4.5 home repair sanding floors with a power sander

06200 4.5 home repair scraping and painting sailboat or powerboat

06205 2.0 home repair sharpening tools

06210 5.0 home repair spreading dirt with a shovel

06220 4.5 home repair washing and waxing hull of sailboat or airplane

06225 2.0 home repair washing and waxing car

06230 4.5 home repair washing fence, painting fence, moderate effort

06240 3.3 home repair wiring, tapping-splicing

CHAPTER 7 – GASTROINTESTINAL SYSTEM

Irritable Bowel Syndrome (IBS) Secondary to Service-Connected Posttraumatic Stress Disorder (PTSD)

Irritable Bowel Syndrome (IBS) is a functional gut disorder that manifests in patients as chronic or recurring abdominal pain, accompanied with alteration of bowel habits. Psychologically, patients presenting with IBS show more depression, emotionality, and worry about their health than do patients without IBS.

Graham et al. in their study *Irritable Bowel Syndrome Symptoms and Health Related Quality of Life in Female Veterans* found that veterans meeting criteria for PTSD represented 51.0% of veterans with IBS symptoms, but only represented 30.9% of veterans without IBS symptoms; a statistical difference.

There are several avenues by which IBS could be linked to PTSD. The pathogenesis of IBS is multifactorial with psychosocial, genetic, nervous system (central and enteric), hormonal, visceral hypersensitivity and infectious/inflammatory components.

Videlock et al. studied the hypothalamic-pituitary-adrenal axis [HPAA] response to a visceral stressor (sigmoidoscopy) in patients with IBS vs. healthy controls and those exposed to early adverse life events (EALs) using salivary cortisol levels. They found higher mean cortisol levels in those who experienced EALs.

Hormones released in response to stress, such as corticotropin-releasing hormone (CRH), regulate changes in gut motility, visceral perception and autonomic function. CRH is released by the hypothalamus and stimulates adrenocorticotropic hormone (ACTH) release by the pituitary gland which in turn stimulates cortisol release from the adrenal cortex.

Exogenous administration of CRH has been shown to increase colonic motility and stimulate serum ACTH with an exaggerated response found in patients with IBS. In a study by Fukudo 10 IBS patients and 10 control subjects underwent pressure transducer placement in the colon and were then injected with CRH. While there was no difference in motility at baseline, the IBS group developed significantly greater colonic motor activity and longer duration of abdominal symptoms in response to CRH administration compared with controls ($P < 0.05$). CRH induced a rise in serum ACTH in both groups, although a significantly higher increase in the IBS group ($P < 0.01$). There was no difference in serum cortisol response in the 2 groups.

Ringel et al. used PET scan to compare cerebral blood flow in patients with IBS and controls with *post-hoc* analyses comparing patients with a history of physical or sexual abuse and patients without abuse. They found a greater increase in anterior cingulate cortex activity in non-IBS subjects and those without a history of abuse. IBS patients showed higher activity in the thalamus, an area previously shown to be associated with pain response.

Psychiatric disturbances are the most frequent comorbidity of visceral pain. Anxiety and depression are the most commonly reported comorbidities.

This complex link between visceral sensation and psychological perceptions are mediated via the brain–gut axis. The brain regions activated in response to colorectal stimulation include the prefrontal cortex (dorsolateral), the insula, the thalamus, the amygdala, and the anterior cingulate cortex (ACC). The amygdala, in particular, the central nucleus of the amygdala (CeA), is a critical region in the limbic system highlighting a clear role of stress pathways in the development of visceral pain. Numerous preclinical studies have shown the important role of the amygdala in pain processing.

Moreover, stress-related changes in bowel habit can attest to the fact that the brain can influence gut function and sensation. Several clinical studies have suggested that psychosocial comorbidity is a major contributor to the severity and impact on quality of life of visceral pain disorders such as IBS and somatic pain disorders such as fibromyalgia. These findings are reinforced by a considerable volume of experimental research that links stress, anxiety, and depression to altered GI sensory and motor function as well as altered pain processing. Indeed, successful management of patients with visceral pain disorders requires careful attention to these psychosocial factors, often in consultation with mental health professionals.

Furthermore, acute stressors such as sexual abuse, rape, traumatic event (near fatal event), and warfare are also risk factors for the development of IBS.

Crohn's Disease

An excerpt from a chapter on Crohn's Disease from Sands & Siegal: Feldman's Textbook of Medicine states (emphasis added):

> "Perianal disease is another common presentation of Crohn's disease. In as many as 24% of patients with Crohn's disease, perianal disease precedes intestinal manifestations, with a mean lead time of four years."

> "Crohn's disease is a condition of chronic inflammation potentially involving any location of the alimentary tract from mouth to anus, but with a propensity for the distal small bowel and proximal large bowel. Inflammation in Crohn's disease often is discontinuous along the longitudinal axis of the intestine and can involve all layers from mucosa to serosa…interspersing of segments of involved bowel with segments of uninvolved bowel. Even within a single biopsy specimen one can see a pronounced variability in the degree of inflammation… Crohn's disease has a predilection for the distal small intestine and proximal colon. One third to one half of all patients have disease affecting both ileum and colon. Another one third have disease confined to the small intestine, primarily the terminal ileum, and there may be an increasing group with isolated colonic disease."

"The typical presenting symptom of colonic disease is diarrhea, occasionally with passage of obvious blood. The severity of the diarrhea tends to correlate with both the extent of colitis and the severity of inflammation, and the presentation may range from minimally altered bowel habits to fulminant colitis. Although most patients with Crohn's colitis have relative or complete sparing of the rectum, proctitis may be the initial presentation in some cases. Among a series of 96 patients with idiopathic proctitis, 13.6% were diagnosed with Crohn's disease, usually within three years of initial presentation…Diarrhea is the most common complaint among patients with Crohn's disease. Increased stool frequency and decreased stool consistency arise through alterations in mucosal function and intestinal motility."

- **Establishing the Diagnosis of Crohn's Disease and Evaluating Disease Activity**

No single symptom, sign, or diagnostic test establishes the diagnosis of Crohn's disease. Rather the diagnosis is established through a total assessment of the clinical presentation with confirmatory evidence from radiologic, endoscopic, and, in most cases, pathologic findings. A rectal examination might disclose findings highly suggestive of the underlying diagnosis or gross or occult blood. Laboratory data may be normal. Ultimately, the diagnosis of Crohn's disease is confirmed by findings on imaging studies, endoscopy, and usually histopathology."

The presentation of Crohn's disease may be subtle and varies considerably. Factors contributing to this variability include the location of disease, the intensity of inflammation, and presence of specific intestinal and extra intestinal complications. Some patients experience symptoms that are mild but long-standing or that are atypical. Such patients are more likely to experience a delay in diagnosis in excess of a year. In the past, a mean delay in diagnosis of 3.3 years from the onset of symptoms was reported, Fecal occult blood may be found in approximately one half of patients.

- **Stress Can be a Contributing Factor in Crohn's Disease**

Research has demonstrated that stress can be a contributing factor in Crohn's disease. Stress and other environmental factors affect both the systemic and local immune status of the intestine. Stress signals are perceived by the central nervous system (CNS), triggering transmission of the signal to the intestine via neuroendocrine mediators. The hypothalamic-pituitary-adrenal axis and the sympathetic-adrenal-medullary axis can modulate secretory, absorption, and barrier functions in the gut.

Crohn's Disease is characterized by increased intestinal permeability and extensive animal research has shown stress significantly influences intestinal permeability. Factors involved in the effects of stress on gut permeability include corticotropin releasing factor (CRF), the autonomic nervous system, and the enteric nervous system. CRF is produced and secreted by the hypothalamus, but has also been found to be secreted in the colonic crypts during times of stress, resulting in increased intestinal permeability. The CNS also influences the degree of intestinal inflammation via the autonomic and enteric nervous systems.

Stress can also contribute to exacerbations of already existing disease. Two prospective studies demonstrated psychological stress, anxiety, and depression are associated with increased Crohn's Disease activity. In one study, 18 Crohn's Disease patients were followed prospectively at 8- to 12-week intervals for two years. Disease activity was measured using the CDAI, Beck Depression Inventory (BDI), and Beck Anxiety Inventory (BAI). The study revealed a strong association between BDI scores and current disease activity when measured simultaneously. Both BDI- and BAI-score increases were independently associated with increased CDAI scores in a subsequent visit 8-12 weeks later.

The second study involved 47 Crohn's Disease patients in remission (after a documented flare) followed for 18 months and assessed using the same scoring inventories as the first study. These researchers also demonstrated psychological stress, anxiety, depression, and altered quality of life were likely to influence CRF.

Fatty Liver

Fatty liver is directly related to the degree of Triglycerides (TG) elevation and results from lipid accumulation within cells of the reticuloendothelial system. Hepatosplenomegaly is rapidly reversible with correction of plasma TG levels.

A research article from the Mayo clinic by Ludwig J, *Nonalcoholic steatohepatitis: Mayo Clinic experiences with a hitherto unnamed disease*, reports how this particular liver disease histologically mimics alcoholic hepatitis, and that it also may progress to cirrhosis. The biopsy specimens from the patients in this study were characterized by the presence of striking fatty changes with evidence of lobular hepatitis, focal necrosis with mixed inflammatory infiltrates, and, in most instances, Mallory bodies; evidence of fibrosis was found in most specimens, and cirrhosis was diagnosed in biopsy tissue from three patients. The presence of hepatomegaly (enlargement of the liver) and mild abnormalities of liver function were common clinical findings.

Mixed Hyperlipidemia, or HLP type 5, has a population prevalence of ~1 in 600. A key distinguishing feature between mixed hyperlipidemia and familial chylomicronemia is the age of onset of presentation. Patients with familial chylomicronemia typically present in childhood or adolescence, whereas mixed hyperlipidemia patients typically present in adulthood. The disease is triggered in patients with an underlying genetic susceptibility coupled with the influence of environmental and hormonal exposures. Signs and symptoms are similar to those seen in familial chylomicronemia, including hepatosplenomegaly, increased pancreatitis risk and some neurological symptoms, such as the inability to concentrate. Epidemiologic evidence links HTG with cardiovascular risk. Therapeutic options such as a fibrates, niacin, and omega-3 fatty acids are recommended to all patients with TG levels exceeding normal values.

Gastroesophageal Reflux Disease (GERD)

GERD can also be rated as analogous to stricture of the esophagus, Diagnostic Code 7203. A 30% evaluation is granted for moderate stricture of the esophagus. A 50% evaluation is warranted for severe stricture of the esophagus, permitting liquids only. An 80% evaluation is warranted for stricture of the esophagus permitting passage of liquids only, with marked impairment of general health. 38 C.F.R. § 4.114, DC 7203. The recurrence rate of cicatricial stenosis of postoperative esophageal diseases is 6–26%. Stenosis of the esophagus seriously affects the patients' quality of life and causes certain complications, including poor nutrition.

7346 Hernia hiatal:	
Symptoms of pain, vomiting, material weight loss and hematemesis or melena with moderate anemia; or other symptom combinations productive of severe impairment of health	60
Persistently recurrent epigastric distress with dysphagia, pyrosis, and regurgitation, accompanied by substernal or arm or shoulder pain, productive of considerable impairment of health	30
With two or more of the symptoms for the 30 % evaluation of less severity	10

7203 Esophagus, stricture of:	
Permitting passage of liquids only, with marked impairment of general health	80
Severe, permitting liquids only	50
Moderate	30

The regulation does not permit combination of Codes 7346 and 7203 because of the rule against pyramiding. Yet, under Code 7346 the rating of 60% provides for EITHER weight loss and hematemesis or melena with moderate anemia, OR other symptom combinations productive of severe impairment of health.

CHAPTER 8 - NEUROLOGY

Traumatic Brain Injury (TBI)

The scientific community has conclusively determined that a person can sustain severe and permanent brain damage even though the trauma to the brain was not marked. Scorza et al. reported:

> "Concussion is a disturbance in brain function caused by direct or indirect force to the head. Terms such as concussion and mild traumatic brain injury are often used interchangeably. It is a functional rather than structural injury that results from shear stress to brain tissue caused by rotational or angular forces—direct impact to the head is not required."

The Third International Conference on Concussion in Sport reported that a concussion may result in neuropathological changes, but the acute clinical symptoms largely reflect a functional disturbance rather than a structural injury. Concussion results in a graded set of clinical symptoms that may or may not involve loss of consciousness; resolution of the clinical and cognitive symptoms typically follows a sequential course; however, it is important to note that in a small percentage of cases, post concussive symptoms may be prolonged. No abnormality on standard structural neuroimaging studies is seen in concussion.

New criteria for evaluating the residuals of TBI under diagnostic code 8045 have been published. The common definition for TBI for the VA and the United States Department of Defense (DoD) is:

> "A traumatically induced structural injury and/or physiological disruption of brain function as a result of an external force that is indicated by new onset or worsening of at least one of the following clinical signs, immediately following the event:
>
> 1) Any period of loss of or a decreased level of consciousness;
> 2) Any loss of memory for events immediately before or after the injury;
> 3) Any alteration in mental state at the time of the injury (confusion, disorientation, slowed thinking, etc.);
> 4) Neurological deficits (weakness, loss of balance, change in vision, praxis, paresis/plegia, sensory loss, aphasia, etc.) that may or may not be transient;
> 5) Intracranial lesion
>
> Any one of these 5 findings is sufficient for a diagnosis."

The mechanisms of injuries that may lead to TBI are many. External forces may include any of the following events: the head being struck by an object, the head striking an object, the brain undergoing an acceleration/deceleration movement without direct external trauma to the head, a foreign body penetrating the brain, forces generated from events such as a blast or explosion, or other force yet to be defined. TBI then may result from a motor vehicle accident, fall, blow to the head, penetrating brain wound, and other types of trauma, both in combat and not in combat, in addition to the blasts/explosions that have been a common source of TBI in veterans of the Afghanistan and Iraq conflicts.

Sequelae of TBI may resolve quickly, within minutes to hours after the neurological event, or they may persist longer. Some sequelae of TBI may be permanent. Most signs and symptoms will manifest immediately following the event. However, other signs and symptoms may be delayed from days to months (e.g., subdural hematoma, seizures, hydrocephalus, spasticity, etc.) Signs and symptoms may occur alone or in varying combinations and may result in a functional impairment. These signs and symptoms are not better explained by pre-existing conditions or other medical, neurological, or psychological causes except in cases of an exacerbation of a pre-existing condition. These generally fall into one or more of the three following categories:

1) Physical: Headache, nausea, vomiting, dizziness, blurred vision, sleep disturbance, weakness, paresis/plegia, sensory loss, spasticity, aphasia, dysphagia, dysarthria, apraxia, balance disorders, disorders of coordination, seizure disorder.
2) Cognitive: Attention, concentration, memory, speed of processing, new learning, planning, reasoning, judgment executive control, self-awareness, language, abstract thinking.
3) Behavioral/emotion: Depression, anxiety, agitation, irritability, impulsivity, aggression.

Note: The signs and symptoms listed above are typical of each category but are not an exhaustive list of all possible signs and symptoms.

These delayed effects of TBI warrant service connection even if they don't appear for days, months, or possibly longer after the trauma, if attributable to an in-service TBI. A medical opinion will be needed in cases where the records do not indicate a clear-cut etiology for a condition that is claimed as a delayed effect.

- **Brain Injury Severity**

The severity of the brain injury is traditionally described as mild, moderate, and severe, based on measures of length of unconsciousness and post-traumatic amnesia. Acute injury severity is determined at the time of the injury, but this severity level, while having some prognostic value, does not necessarily reflect the patient's ultimate level of functioning. It is recognized that serial assessments of the patient's cognitive, emotional, behavioral and social functioning are required. This means that a veteran who was initially designated as having mild TBI may have severe residuals, and one who was designated as having severe TBI may have only mild residuals. Thus, the severity level assigned at the time of the acute trauma should not be a factor in determining the evaluation. Classification of the acute level of severity has no bearing on C&P evaluations.

Determination of severity is made at the time of the injury, that is, it is a determination of acute injury severity. Once this acute level of severity is determined, it does not change, regardless of the veteran's course or

extent of residuals. The patient is classified as mild/moderate/severe if he or she meets criteria in more than one category of severity, the higher severity level is assigned. If it is not clinically possible to determine the brain injury level of severity because of medical complications (e.g., medically induced coma), other severity markers are required to make a determination of the severity of the brain injury. It is also recognized that the symptoms associated with PTSD may overlap with symptoms of mild traumatic brain injury. Differential diagnosis of brain injury and PTSD is required for accurate diagnosis and treatment.
Note: this stratification does not apply to penetrating brain injuries where the dura mater is breached.

LOC – Loss of consciousness
AOC – Alteration of consciousness/mental state
PTA – Post-traumatic amnesia
GCA – Glasgow Coma Scale (measured at or after 24 hours)

MILD: Normal structural imaging
LOC = 0-30 min
AOC = a moment up to 24 hrs.
PTA = 0-1 day
GCS = 13-15

MODERATE: Normal or abnormal structural imaging
LOC > 30 min and < 24 hours
AOC > 24 hours, severity based on other criteria
PTA > 1 and < 7 days
GCS = 9-12

(Note: PTA > 7 days & GCS = 3-8 are also mentioned partially under moderate going to severe)

SEVERE: Normal or abnormal structural imaging
LOC > 24 hours
AOC > 24 hours, severity based on other criteria
PTA > 7 days
GCS = 3-8

Regarding testing for brain injury, the trauma may or may not cause structural damage, and thus, may not be detected by traditional imaging studies such as MRI or CT. Traumas that produce more subtle damage that manifests by altered brain function, may be identified by other imaging techniques such as functional MRI, diffusion tensor imaging, positron emission tomography (PET) scanning, as well as electrophysiological testing such as electroencephalography. These may be used to detect damage to or physiological alteration of brain function. In addition, altered brain function may manifest by altered performance on neuropsychological or other standardized testing of function.

- **TBI Residuals**

TBI residuals may be physical, cognitive and behavioral/emotional. Some of these residuals can be rated under the criteria in diagnostic code 8045; others will require evaluation under the diagnostic codes in the neurologic system, as well as under diagnostic codes in the mental disorders, eye, audio, and other body systems.

Physical residuals – should be evaluated under the most appropriate diagnostic code and body system and combined under §4.25 may include:

- Motor and sensory dysfunction, including pain, of the extremities and face
- Visual impairment
- Hearing loss and tinnitus
- Loss of sense of smell and taste
- Seizures
- Gait, coordination, and balance problems
- Speech and other communication difficulties, including aphasia and related disorders, and dysarthria
- Neurogenic bladder
- Neurogenic bowel
- Cranial nerve dysfunctions
- Autonomic nerve dysfunctions
- Endocrine dysfunctions

Behavioral/emotional dysfunction – can result from a TBI, but comorbid mental disorders (especially depression, PTSD, and anxiety) are common in veterans with TBI. In some cases, TBI and one or more comorbid mental disorders both result in behavioral/emotional symptoms in the same veteran. The etiology of the behavioral/emotional dysfunction must be determined by the examiner. If it is impossible to make such a determination without speculation, then that should be stated. Behavioral emotional symptoms due to TBI fall most often under the neurobehavioral symptoms facet of the table in diagnostic code 8045, but at times (such as when mild anxiety is a major symptom) may also fall under the subjective symptoms facet.

Special Monthly Compensation (SMC): Revised diagnostic code 8045 points out the importance of considering the need for special monthly compensation for such problems as loss of use of an extremity, certain sensory impairments, erectile dysfunction, the need for aid and attendance (including for protection from hazards or dangers incident to the daily environment due to cognitive impairment), being housebound, etc.

Combining under §4.25/avoidance of pyramiding. Each residual condition should be evaluated separately as long as the same signs and symptoms are not used to support more than one evaluation. Then combine the evaluations under §4.25.

Evaluate a recently discharged veteran for prestabilization ratings based on § 4.28.

Posttraumatic Headaches

Posttraumatic headaches (PTH) are common in the TBI population, with a prevalence ranging from 30 to 90% depending on the type of measurement instrument administered to patients. Posttraumatic headaches may persist long after the TBI, with 18% to 22% of PTH sufferers still experiencing symptoms one year later.

Approximately 75% of the 1.7 million patients with traumatic head injuries in the United States (annual) are classified as mild. Posttraumatic headaches in this population may be the major cause of persistent disability. Posttraumatic migraine sufferers are reported to have longer recovery times from mild TBI than other PTH patients. In one study, patients suffering from posttraumatic migraines demonstrated a 7.3 times greater risk for extended recovery time than nonmigraine TBI patients. Disability is a key factor in planning level of care based on the patient's work and family obligations.

Migraine is a common, multifactorial, disabling, recurrent, hereditary neurovascular headache disorder. It usually strikes sufferers a few times per year in childhood and then progresses to a few times per week in adulthood, particularly in females. Attacks often begin with warning signs (prodromes) and aura (transient focal neurological symptoms) whose origin is thought to involve the hypothalamus, brainstem, and cortex.

Once the headache develops, it typically throbs, intensifies with an increase in intracranial pressure, and presents itself in association with nausea, vomiting, and abnormal sensitivity to light, noise, and smell. It can also be accompanied by abnormal skin sensitivity (allodynia) and muscle tenderness. Collectively, the symptoms that accompany migraine from the prodromal stage through the headache phase suggest that multiple neuronal systems function abnormally. Callaghan et al. reported:

> "Post-traumatic headache (PTH), a headache attributed to head and/or neck trauma, is the commonest Secondary headache with the prevalence of chronic PTH varying from 3.2% to

6.8% in children with head injury. The most common headache types recognized are episodic tension type headache and migraine without aura. Severity of head injury has not been found to correlate with severity or duration of PTH.

The pathophysiology of CPTH is not well elucidated, with a variety of mechanisms proposed including anatomical and physiological changes (degeneration of nerve fibres, reduced regional cerebral blood flow, diffuse axonal injury at grey white matter interface); abnormalities in calcium and magnesium homeostasis, cerebral metabolic activities, endogenous opiates and serotonin; neurochemical changes (excessive release of excitatory neurotransmitters glutamate, aspartate, acetylcholine leading to secondary neuronal damage and delayed onset neurological lesion)."

Tinnitus

Even when tinnitus and hearing loss occur after military service, it does not rule out that the noise trauma did occur during military service. The Institute of Medicine was asked by the Veterans' Administration to investigate this very question. The following are excerpts from a report by the Institute of Medicine that looked at the question of how to assess tinnitus in veterans and whether or not tinnitus can appear in a delayed fashion:

"Tinnitus is a perceived sound that cannot be attributed to an external sound source (Eggermont, 2003). It is a subjective phenomenon, perceivable only by the person who is experiencing it. The Institute of Medicine committee was asked to review the evidence regarding noise levels that can cause tinnitus and other risk factors for tinnitus. Some studies define persistent or prolonged tinnitus as lasting at least 5 minutes (e.g., Coles, 1984; Parving, et al., 1993; Palmer, et al., 2002; Sindhusake, et al, 2003b). Persistent tinnitus can be perceived continuously (all or most of the time) or occasionally. A given episode of tinnitus may also resolve, with new episodes possible in the future.

Tinnitus is considered a symptom rather than an illness (NRC, 1982). It is associated with many conditions, including noise exposure and noise-induced hearing loss. It is not always possible to identify a precipitating cause of tinnitus. A survey of tinnitus patients found that only 54% attributed their tinnitus to a particular cause (Stouffer and Tyler, 1990). The onset of tinnitus is described by some as gradual and by others as sudden (Axelsson and Barrenas, 1992). In a population-based study of older adults, 55% of participants with tinnitus reported a gradual onset, 24% reported a sudden onset, and the remainder did not know (Sindhusake et al., 2003b). Uncertainty about the onset of tinnitus can make the identification of a precipitating cause challenging.

Individuals differ in their susceptibility and reaction to tinnitus. The mechanisms underlying tinnitus are not completely understood. Generally, it is reasonable to presume that the involvement of central components of the auditory system "results in" the perception of sound. In addition, if there is an emotional reaction to the tinnitus, other areas of the central nervous system that are involved in emotionally charged events, such as the amygdala, are activated. The IOM determined that the onset of noise-induced tinnitus might be delayed because studies in laboratory animals have shown that degenerative processes initiated by the noise exposure continue in central auditory pathways after termination of the exposure (Kim et al., 1997; Morest, et al., 1998). Although degenerative changes in afferent pathways will most likely not affect auditory thresholds, it is possible that they could contribute to other central processes such as tinnitus. 'The time required for this reorganization might vary across individuals and potentially could be a long-term process.'"

CHAPTER 9 - RHEUMATOLOGY

Chronic Fatigue Syndrome and Fibromyalgia

§ 4.88a Chronic fatigue syndrome. [59 FR 60902, Nov. 29, 1994]

(a) For VA purposes, the diagnosis of chronic fatigue syndrome requires:
    (1) new onset of debilitating fatigue severe enough to reduce daily activity to less than 50% of the usual level for at least six months; and
    (2) the exclusion, by history, physical examination, and laboratory tests, of all other clinical conditions that may produce similar symptoms; and
    (3) six or more of the following:
        (i) acute onset of the condition,
        (ii) low grade fever,
        (iii) non-exudative pharyngitis,
        (iv) palpable or tender cervical or axillary lymph nodes,
        (v) generalized muscle aches or weakness,
        (vi) fatigue lasting 24 hours or longer after exercise,
        (vii) headaches (of a type, severity, or pattern that is different from headaches in the pre-morbid state),
        (viii) migratory joint pains,
        (ix) neuropsychologic symptoms,
        (x) sleep disturbance

Fibromyalgia syndrome (FMS) is a common and distressful condition with multiple multiple facets. FMS patients can be subclassified into five groups based on their clinical presentations:

- Predominant pain and fatigue;
- Predominant anxiety, stress, and depression;
- Predominant multiple sites of pain complaints and tender points (TP);
- Predominant numbness and swollen feeling;
- Associated features, that is, irritable bowel syndrome and headaches.

Fatigue is the hallmark of the chronic fatigue syndrome (CFS); fatigue must be new, persistent, or relapsing and associated with a 50% reduction in a patient's premorbid activity for at least 6 months. In the mid-1980s, reports erroneously linked CFS to Epstein-Barr virus (EBV), and CFS continues to be controversial.

Fibromyalgia is a similar disorder of widespread musculoskeletal pain and fatigue with other symptoms, such as poor sleep. CFS and fibromyalgia are overlapping disorders; about 75% of patients with CFS also meet the criteria for fibromyalgia, and vice versa. The onset of CFS is often acute after an infectious illness, typically viral, whereas the onset is often gradual with fibromyalgia.

The cause of CFS and Fibromyalgia are unknown. Patients with fibromyalgia report either a gradual onset of their disorder or an "event," such as a flulike illness or physical trauma. Patients with CFS often recall the onset after an acute viral illness. The cardinal symptom of CFS is fatigue. The fatigue of CFS refers to a state of profound mental and physical exhaustion that cannot be explained by ongoing exertion or activities. The fatigue also is disproportionately exacerbated by activity and is not ameliorated by rest. Other characteristic symptoms of CFS include self-perceived impairments of short-term memory and concentration, sleep problems, muscle and joint pain, headache, dizziness, allergic symptoms, and depression.

In 1990 the American College of Rheumatology outlined guidelines for diagnosing Fibromyalgia by requiring that widespread pain be present for 3 months or more. Widespread pain refers to pain involving both sides of the body and above and below the waist. In addition, to fulfill the diagnostic criteria, pain must be present in 11 or more of 18 specified tender points on digital palpation. Other symptoms and signs include sleep problems, fatigue, stiffness, and cold intolerance.

The CDC case definition is currently the most accepted basis for diagnosing CFS. A patient must have unexplained persistent fatigue for 6 months that is new and not caused by exertion:

1. Clinically evaluated, unexplained, persistent, or relapsing fatigue for at least 6 months that:

    - Is of new or definite onset,
    - Is not the result of ongoing exertion,
    - Is not substantially alleviated by rest, and,

- Results in substantial reduction in previous levels of activities.

2. Four or more of the following concurrent symptoms on a persistent or recurrent basis during 6 or more consecutive months of illness, none of which may predate the fatigue:

- Self-reported impairment in short-term memory or concentration that is severe enough to cause substantial reduction in previous levels of occupational, educational, social, or personal activities previous levels of occupational, educational, social, or personal activities,
- Sore throat,
- Tender cervical or axillary lymph nodes,
- Muscle pain,
- Multijoint pain without joint swelling or redness,
- Headaches of a new type, pattern, or severity,
- Unrefreshing sleep,
- Postexertional malaise lasting more than 24 hours.

The diagnosis of CFS is difficult and remains one of exclusion. No laboratory test can confirm the diagnosis; routine laboratory tests are normal, and the erythrocyte sedimentation rate is not elevated. Similarly, antinuclear antibody or rheumatoid factor testing should be ordered only if the patient has joint complaints. Selected immunologic tests may be abnormal in patients with

CFS but are indicated only for research purposes. Although symptoms of the so-called yeast connection or Candida hypersensitivity syndrome overlap those of CFS, no evidence indicates that the "yeast syndrome" exists, and testing for Candida antibodies is not indicated.

Cortisol excretion is decreased in CFS patients compared with controls. This may result from a deficiency of corticotropin-releasing hormone (CRH) or another stimulus of the pituitary-adrenal axis. In contrast to patients with CFS, cortisol secretion may be increased in patients with primary depression.

CFS has been associated with neurally mediated low blood pressure. In one study 30% to 89% of patients with CFS dropped their blood pressure when placed on a tilt table and responded to salt loading, fludrocortisone, beta-adrenergic blockers, and disopyramide.

Magnetic resonance imaging (MRI) brain scans may show multiple foci of high signal intensity in the white matter in patients with CFS compared with controls. The meaning of these findings is unknown, and an MRI brain scan is not useful as a diagnostic test.

Patients complain of multiple cognitive defects, but various neuropsychologic tests have not been of value in documenting these abnormalities. Although fatigue is a hallmark of CFS, no myopathy has been identified. Similarly, patients often complain of weakness but on testing demonstrate normal muscle strength.

Roizenblatt et al. reported that FMS patients with phasic alpha sleep reported significantly more pain and more tender points following their disturbed sleep. Yunus et al. showed that poor sleep is significantly ($P = 0.01$ or less) correlated with all important fibromyalgia features, e.g., pain, number of pain sites, fatigue, global severity, functional status by Health Assessment Questionnaire (HAQ), as well as anxiety, depression, and stress (as measured by validated questionnaires).

Widespread pain and multiple tender points are characteristic of fibromyalgia, but again, no diagnostic laboratory test exists. Patients with fibromyalgia sleep poorly, and sleep abnormalities have been identified on electroencephalograms; however, these findings are not specific for fibromyalgia.

Neuroendocrine abnormalities, such as reduced excretion of urinary free cortisol and decreased levels of insulin growth were reported.

Many patients with FM complain of cognitive difficulties. A recent study has shown poorer working memory, word groping, and poorer vocabulary in FMS as compared with age-matched controls. While no appropriate studies have been published, these symptoms may be contributed by poor sleep, fatigue, psychologic factors, and medications among clinic patients.

On May 11, 1998, Deputy Commissioner for Disability and Income Security Programs, Susan Daniels, wrote a memoranda to an ALJ who argued that the symptoms of

FM should not be considered medically acceptable without clinical and laboratory diagnostic techniques in support of the claimant's application for disability determination:

> "Your letter states that fibromyalgia and CFS do not constitute medically determinable impairments within the meaning of section 223(d)(3) of the Social Security Act because there are no acceptable medical criteria by which these impairments can be diagnosed.... However, SSA has taken a definitive position that fibromyalgia and CFS can constitute medically determinable impairments within the meaning of the statute. As you noted in your letter, CFS was discussed in the process unification training in 1996-1997...This position is consistent with the instructions in Program Operations Manual System (POMS) DI 24515.075, Disability Digest No. 93-5, and Social Security Rulings (SSRs) 96-3p, 96-4p, and 96-7p, issued on July 2, 1996, which detail our policies as to how symptoms affect determinations of the presence of a medically determinable impairment, impairment severity, and the ability to engage in sustained work activity."

In a report issued February 2015, the Committee of the Institute of Medicine stated:

> "Myalgic encephalomyelitis (ME) and chronic fatigue syndrome (CFS) are serious, debilitating conditions that affect millions of people in the

United States and around the world. ME/CFS can cause significant impairment and disability. Despite substantial efforts by researchers to better understand ME/CFS, there is no known cause or effective treatment. Diagnosing the disease remains a challenge, and patients often struggle with their illness for years before an identification is made. Some health care providers have been skeptical about the serious physiological - rather than psychological - nature of the illness. Once diagnosed, patients often complain of receiving hostility from their health care provider as well as being subjected to treatment strategies that exacerbate their symptoms.

Beyond Myalgic Encephalomyelitis/Chronic Fatigue Syndrome proposes new diagnostic clinical criteria for ME/CFS and a new term for the illness - systemic exertion intolerance disease (SEID). According to this report, the term myalgic encephalomyelitis does not accurately describe this illness, and the term chronic fatigue syndrome can result in trivialization and stigmatization for patients afflicted with this illness.

Beyond Myalgic/Encephalomyelitis Chronic Fatigue Syndrome stresses that SEID is a medical - not a psychiatric or psychological - illness. This report lists the major symptoms of SEID and recommends a diagnostic process. One of the report's most important conclusions is that a thorough history, physical examination, and targeted work-up are necessary and often sufficient for diagnosis. The new criteria will allow a large percentage of undiagnosed patients to receive an accurate diagnosis and appropriate care.

Beyond Myalgic Encephalomyelitis/Chronic Fatigue Syndrome will be a valuable resource to promote the prompt diagnosis of patients with this complex, multisystem, and often devastating disorder; enhance public understanding; and provide a firm foundation for future improvements in diagnosis and treatment."

5025 Fibromyalgia (fibrositis, primary fibromyalgia syndrome)	
With widespread musculoskeletal pain and tender points, with or without associated fatigue, sleep disturbance, stiffness, paresthesias, headache, irritable bowel symptoms, depression, anxiety, or Raynaud's-like symptoms:	
That are constant, or nearly so, and refractory to therapy	40
That are episodic, with exacerbations often precipitated by environmental or emotional stress or by overexertion, but that are present more than one-third of the time	20
That require continuous medication for control	10

> Note: Widespread pain means pain in both the left and right sides of the body, that is both above and below the waist, and that affects both the axial skeleton (*i.e.*, cervical spine, anterior chest, thoracic spine, or low back) and the extremities.

Systemic Lupus Erythematosus

After excluding alternative diagnoses, Rheumatologists diagnose Systemic Lupus Erythematosus (SLE) in patients who fulfill the 1997 American College of Rheumatology (ACR) criteria; a patient must satisfy at least 4 of 13 criteria.

Expanded list of SLE features:

1. Rash (incl. butterfly, livedo reticularis, vasculitis)
2. Discoid lupus
3. Raynaud's phenomenon
4. Alopecia
5. Photosensitivity
6. Oral/nasal ulceration
7. Arthritis
8. DNA-bc > 40U/ml
9. False + ve syphilis serology
10. Albustix + +
11. Granular urinary casts
12. Pleurisy/pericarditis
13. Neuropsychiatric disorder
14. Cytopenia

15. Fever
16. Ocular disease

- **Antinuclear Antibody Test**

The American rheumatological society reported that only about 11-13% of persons with a positive ANA test have lupus and up to 15% of completely healthy people have a positive ANA test. Thus, a positive ANA test does not automatically translate into a diagnosis of lupus or any autoimmune or connective tissue disease.

ANA-negative SLE has been recognized since the 1970s, often due to inaccurate methodology used before 1990. Other factors that may also influence ANA negativity in SLE patients include disease duration and treatment exposure. The frequency of ANA-negative SLE is higher in patients presenting at an early stage of their disease. In addition, SLE patients who have longstanding disease and/or have undergone treatment may lose ANA reactivity and become serologically negative over time.
It is uniformly accepted that ANA-negative SLE seems to be a subgroup of SLE that has not previously been given adequate attention. Antinuclear antibody-negative SLE has been implied, if not directly considered, in many studies of SLE over the years. Two series citing ten and eight cases, respectively, of ANA-negative SLE have drawn more direct attention to this entity and Maddison et al. presented data on 66 cases of SLE with serological abnormalities but negative ANA tests. In each study the cases were collected over a number of

years as being atypical members of larger series of ANA-positive lupus.

Fessel et al. reported 16 patients with four or more features, and a further six each with three features who were diagnosed as ANA negative SLE. It remains to be seen how large the ANA-negative SLE group will become once it is actively sought. The prevalence of SLE is not known but using a suggested figure of one in 2000, the study half-million catchment population should contain around 250 cases of SLE. The 22 ANA-negative cases detected to date would represent 8-9%. The author noted that the diagnosis of SLE is often difficult; only seven of his 22 cases had been diagnosed by their attending physician.

Bohan et al. reported 5 well-studied patients with SLE who initially presented with negative serology despite active multisystemic disease. When followed from 10 months to 7 years, negative serologic markers, including the ANA, LE cell test, and anti-DNA, were seen to change from negative to positive, analogous to the seronegative rheumatoid patient who may become seropositive.

Frequency of Signs and Symptoms of Systemic Lupus Erythematosus

Signs and symptoms	% at onset	% at anytime
Fatigue	50	74 to 100
Fever	36	40 to 80 +
Weight loss	21	44 to 60 +
Arthritis or arthralgia	62 to 67	83 to 95
Skin	73	80 to 91
Butterfly rash	28 to 38	48 to 54
Photosensitivity	29	41 to 60
Mucous membrane lesion	10 to 21	27 to 52
Alopecia	32	18 to 71
Raynaud's phenomenon	17 to 33	22 to 71
Purpura	10	15 to 34
Urticaria	1	4 to 8
Renal	16 to 38	34 to 73
Nephrosis	5	11 to 18
Gastrointestinal	18	38 to 44
Pulmonary	2 to 12	24 to 98
Pleurisy	17	30 to 45

Effusion		24
Pneumonia		29
Cardiac	15	20 to 46
Pericarditis	8	8 to 48
Murmurs		23
ECG changes		34 to 70
Lymphadenopathy	7 to 16	21 to 50
Splenomegaly	5	9 to 20
Hepatomegaly	2	7 to 25
Central nervous system	12 to 21	25 to 75
Functional		Most
Psychosis	1	5 to 52
Convulsions	0.5	2 to 20

Adapted from: Von Feldt JM, Postgrad Med 1995; 97:79. Graphic 70386 Version 4.0 ACR criteria for the classification of systemic lupus erythematosus.

Rheumatoid Arthritis

5002 Arthritis rheumatoid (atrophic) As an active process:	
With constitutional manifestations associated with active joint involvement, totally incapacitating	
Less than criteria for 100% but with weight loss and anemia productive of severe impairment of health or severely incapacitating exacerbations occurring 4 or more times a year or a lesser number over prolonged periods	
Symptom combinations productive of definite impairment of health objectively supported by examination findings or incapacitating exacerbations occurring 3 or more times a year	
One or two exacerbations a year in a well-established diagnosis	

BVA 9404900 DOCKET NO. 91-43 196:

> "The rating schedule provides that rheumatoid arthritis as an active process will be assigned a 100% rating with constitutional manifestations associated with active joint involvement that is totally incapacitating.
>
> A 60% rating is assigned when the symptoms are less than the criteria for a 100% rating but with weight loss and anemia productive of severe impairment of health or severely incapacitating

exacerbations occurring 4 or more time a year or a lesser number over prolonged periods.

A 40% rating is warranted where there are symptom combinations productive of definite impairment of health objectively supported by examination findings or incapacitating exacerbations occurring 3 or more times a year. One or two exacerbations a year in a well-established diagnosis would warrant a 20% evaluation. Chronic residuals such as limitation of motion are rated under the appropriate diagnostic codes for the specific joints involved. Where the limitation of motion of the specific joint or joints involved is noncompensable a 10% rating is applicable for each such major joint or group of minor joints affected by limitation of motion, to be combined, not added under diagnostic code 5002. The ratings for the active process will not be combined with the residual ratings for limitation of motion or ankylosis. Rather, the higher evaluation will be assigned. 38 C.F.R. Part 4, Code 5002 (1992)"

Rheumatoid arthritis is a chronic systemic inflammatory disease characterized by joint destruction. It affects 0.03% to 1.5% of the population worldwide. Its incidence peaks between the ages of 35 and 45 years; however, the age-related prevalence continues to increase even after age 65. It occurs 3 times more frequently in women than men. The cause remains unknown. The presentation of an unknown antigen to genetically susceptible persons is believed to trigger rheumatoid arthritis.

- **Pathogenesis of Rheumatoid Arthritis**

There is an immunogenetic predisposition to the development of rheumatoid arthritis. Class II major histocompatibility complex molecules on the surface of antigen-presenting cells are responsible for initiating cellular immune responses and for stimulating the differentiation of B lymphocytes into plasma cells that produce antibody.

The immune reaction begins in the synovial lining of the joint. The earliest pathologic changes in the disease are microvascular injury that increases vascular permeability and the accumulation of inflammatory cells (CD4+ lymphocytes, polymorphonuclear leukocytes, and plasma cells) in the perivascular space.

Pro-inflammatory cytokines are released. Mediators of inflammation promote synovial angiogenesis and synovial cell proliferation. The local inflammatory response becomes self-perpetuating. Cytokines continue to play an important role, including tumor necrosis factor-α, interleukin-1, and interleukin-6. Proliferating synovium of activated macrophages and fibroblasts polarizes into a centripetally invasive pannus, destroying the weakened cartilage and subchondral bone. Chondrocytes, stimulated in the inflammatory milieu, release their own proteases and collagenases.

Patients have swelling, pain, and joint stiffness with the onset of vascular injury of the synovial lining, angiogenesis, and cellular proliferation. Joint warmth, swelling, pain, and limitation of motion worsen as the synovial membrane proliferates and the inflammatory reaction builds. Histologic and radiographic evidence of rheumatoid synovitis is found in clinically unaffected joints, suggesting that the disease may be present for a period of time before clinical manifestations appear.

Clinical Features of Rheumatoid Arthritis

The joints most commonly involved (more than 85% of patients) in rheumatoid arthritis are the metacarpophalangeal, proximal interphalangeal, wrist, and metatarsophalangeal joints. The distal interphalangeal joints are typically spared. The distribution of involvement is symmetric and polyarticular (five or more joints); predominantly, small joints are involved. Ultimately, the knees (80% of patients), ankles (80%), shoulders (60%), elbows (50%), hips (50%), acromioclavicular joints (50%), atlantoaxial joint (50%), and temporomandibular joints (30%) can be involved.

Joints affected with rheumatoid arthritis are warm and swollen. The joint enlargement feels spongy and occurs with the thickening of the synovium. An associated joint effusion may make the joint feel fluctuant. Patients describe deep aching and soreness in the involved joints, which are aggravated by use and can be present at rest. Prolonged morning joint stiffness and "gelling" throughout the body and recurrence of this stiffness after resting are some of the many constitutional features that complicate rheumatoid arthritis.

Constitutional Features of Rheumatoid Arthritis
- Fatigue, weight loss, muscle pain, excessive sweating, or low-grade fever may be reported by patients presenting with rheumatoid arthritis.
- **Carpal Tunnel Syndrome in Rheumatoid Arthritis**

Rheumatoid arthritis is a common cause of carpal tunnel syndrome (pregnancy is the commonest cause). The sudden appearance of bilateral carpal tunnel syndrome should raise the question of an early inflammatory arthritis. This syndrome is associated with paresthesias of the hand in a typical median nerve distribution. Discomfort may radiate up the forearm or into the upper arm. The symptoms worsen with prolonged flexion of the wrist and at night. Late complications include thenar muscle weakness and atrophy and permanent sensory loss. Treatment includes resting splints, control of inflammation, and local injection of glucocorticosteroid. Surgical release is recommended for persistent symptoms.

CHAPTER 10 – ENDOCRINOLOGY
Diabetes Mellitus - Etiology and Classification

Diabetes mellitus is a metabolic disorder characterized by increased fasting and postprandial concentrations of glucose. It is the commonest metabolic disorder and affects about 10% of the U.S. population. The classification of this disorder into two broad categories is somewhat artificial and a degree of overlap exists.

Type 1 diabetes mellitus (T1D) is characterized by immune destruction of the insulin-producing beta cells in the islets of Langerhans. It affects 10% to 20% of the diabetic population and usually appears at a younger age. Most patients eventually lose all endogenous insulin secretion and are prone to the development of ketoacidosis.

Type 2 diabetes (T2D) is characterized by defective insulin secretion and action. Environmental factors such as obesity have an important role in the development of T2D. T2D can occur at any age. T2D usually has an insidious onset. Often, the disease is diagnosed during routine laboratory testing by the presence of glycosuria or fasting hyperglycemia. Patients may complain of blurring of vision, myopia, episodes of recurrent skin infections, or monilial vaginitis (females) or balanitis (males). Occasionally, patients may present with evidence of chronic diabetic complications (neuropathy, nephropathy, or retinopathy) but without symptoms related to glucose intolerance).

(Mayo Clinic Internal Medicine Concise Textbook (Page 204). CRC Press.)

- **Diagnosis of Diabetes Mellitus**

The normal fasting plasma glucose concentration is less than 105 mg/dL. In adults (but not pregnant women), fasting values of 126 mg/dL or greater on two or more occasions confirm the diagnosis of diabetes mellitus.

Fasting values between 110 mg/dL and 125 mg/dL encompass the class of impaired fasting glucose. In July 1997, the American Diabetes Association recommended lowering the level for diagnosis from 140 mg/dL to 126 mg/dL because epidemiologic data demonstrated a progressive increase in microvascular complications with progressive impairment in fasting glucose concentrations greater than 105 mg/dL.

The following table provides the percentages that indicate diagnoses of normal, diabetes, and prediabetes according to A1C levels:

Diagnosis	A1C Level
Normal	below 5.7 %
Diabetes	6.5 % or above
Prediabetes	5.7 to 6.4 %

Having prediabetes is a risk factor for getting type 2 diabetes. People with prediabetes may be retested each year. Within the prediabetes A1C range of 5.7 to 6.4 %, the higher the A1C, the greater the risk of diabetes. Those with prediabetes are likely to develop type 2 diabetes within 10 years.

7913 Diabetes mellitus	
Requiring more than one daily injection of insulin, restricted diet, and regulation of activities (avoidance of strenuous occupational and recreational activities) with episodes of ketoacidosis or hypoglycemic reactions requiring at least three hospitalizations per year or weekly visits to a diabetic care provider, plus either progressive loss of weight and strength or complications that would be compensable if separately evaluated	100
Requiring insulin, restricted diet, and regulation of activities with episodes of ketoacidosis or hypoglycemic reactions requiring one or two hospitalizations per year or twice a month visits to a diabetic care provider, plus complications that would not be compensable if separately evaluated	60
Requiring insulin, restricted diet, and regulation of activities	40
Requiring insulin and restricted diet, or; oral hypoglycemic agent and restricted diet	20

- **BVA Decision Regarding Service Connection for Diabetes Mellitus**

DOCKET NO. DATE 12 - 33 038 07 July 2015

"The Veteran contends that his current type 2 diabetes mellitus condition had its onset during service. Specifically, he contends that his in-service diagnosis of impaired glucose tolerance was incorrect, and should have been a diagnosis of diabetes mellitus, as his blood sugar level was noted.

The Veteran's February 1969 induction physical examination and February 1971 separation physical examination reports are negative for complaints, treatment, or a diagnosis of diabetes mellitus or an impaired glucose condition. However, a January 1970 service treatment record indicates glucose.

A record indicates glucose of 120. A May 19 record indicates a probable diagnosis of impaired glucose tolerance versus diabetes mellitus. A subsequent June 19 record indicates glucose of.

Post-service private treatment records indicate a diagnosis of borderline diabetes mellitus in December 19 and a diagnosis of diabetes mellitus in November 2009. Subsequent VA outpatient treatment records demonstrate diagnoses of type 2 diabetes mellitus, and the Veteran has continued to seek treatment for his condition.

The examiner opined that the cause of the Veteran's type 2 diabetes could not be determined. The examiner did, however, report that it appeared that the Veteran had impaired glucose tolerance during service or impaired fasting glucose based on fasting blood sugar within the range of 100 to 125 mg/dl. The examiner reported that this could be considered prediabetes, which increases the risk of developing type 2 diabetes. The examiner noted that the natural history of impaired fasting glucose and impaired glucose tolerance was considered to be variable. In this regard, the examiner cited an article by medical practitioners in the field, indicating that approximately 25% of subjects with either will progress to diabetes over three to five years, and subjects with additional diabetes risk factors including obesity and family history are more likely to develop diabetes.

The examiner further reported that the Veteran appeared to have a prediabetic condition or prediabetes noted in his records during service. He further stated that prediabetes, impaired glucose tolerance, or impaired fasting glucose were strong risk factors for developing overt type 2 diabetes.
Regarding the Veteran, the examiner reported that he had other risk factors including family history and weight.

The examiner stated that prevention of the progression to type 2 diabetes sometimes can be successful; however, in this case, the Veteran did go on to develop overt type 2 diabetes. The examiner concluded that although he could not determine the cause of the Veteran's type 2 diabetes, his disease could be considered as a progression from prediabetes."

- **Inhaled Corticosteroids and the Risk of Diabetes Onset and Progression**

Samy Suissa, Ph.D. et al. reported that the use of inhaled corticosteroids is associated with a significant 34% increase in the risk of incident diabetes. This risk increased with higher doses of inhaled corticosteroids, Moreover, in patients already treated for diabetes with oral hypoglycemic agents, the risk of progression to insulin also increased by 34% with the use of inhaled corticosteroids, with the higher doses associated with a 54% increase in this risk.

Clearly, systemic corticosteroids are associated with insulin resistance and hyperglycemia. Therefore, it is not surprising that inhaled corticosteroids, especially at high doses with clear systemic effects, might result in hyperglycemia and an earlier need for therapy or its intensification.

- **Diabetes and Renal Failure**

The incidence and prevalence of diabetes mellitus have grown significantly throughout the world, due primarily to the increase in type 2 diabetes. This increase in the number of people developing diabetes has had a major impact on the development of diabetic kidney disease (DKD).

DKD remains one of the most frequent complications of both types of diabetes, and diabetes is the leading cause of end-stage renal disease (ESRD), accounting for approximately 50% of cases in the developed world. Although incidence rates for ESRD attributable to DKD have stabilized over the past few years, differences remain among high-risk subgroups. Middle-aged African Americans, Native Americans, and Hispanics continue to have higher rates of ESRD. These disparities in health care may be linked, in part, to the increasing rates of obesity and type 2 diabetes in youth, which disproportionately occur in these populations and allow for the development of diabetes complications earlier in life.

Albuminuria is a marker for kidney/glomerular disease as well as for CVD risk and is often the first clinical indicator of the presence of DKD. It is a clinically useful tool for predicting prognosis and for monitoring response to therapy. Despite the strength of albuminuria as a risk biomarker for DKD and CVD outcomes, there are considerable limitations. Importantly, not all people with DKD and reduced eGFR have increased albuminuria.

In the UK, Prospective Diabetes Study (UKPDS), 51% of those who developed an estimated creatinine clearance of <60 mL/min/1.73 m^2 ever tested positive for albuminuria. Some, but not all, observational studies show that the rate of loss of GFR is slower in those type 2 diabetic patients with low or normal albuminuria.

- **Hypertension and Diabetes Mellitus**

Diabetes mellitus and hypertension are interrelated diseases that strongly predispose an individual to atherosclerotic cardiovascular disease. Hypertension is about twice as frequent in individuals with diabetes as in those without. The prevalence of coexisting hypertension and diabetes appears to be increasing in industrialized nations because populations are aging and both hypertension and NIDDM incidence increases with age.

Data obtained from death certificates show that hypertensive disease has been implicated in 4.4% of deaths coded to diabetes, and diabetes was involved in 10% of deaths coded to hypertensive disease. Indeed, an estimated 35% to 75% of diabetic cardiovascular and renal complications can be attributed to hypertension.

Hypertension also contributes to diabetic retinopathy, which is the leading cause of newly diagnosed blindness in the United States. For all these reasons, hypertension and diabetes should be recognized and treated early and aggressively.

Many anatomic and functional abnormalities of the vascular endothelium are associated with both diabetes mellitus and hypertension. In insulin-resistant states, endothelial cell lipoprotein lipase activity is decreased, as is the conversion of cholesterol ester–enriched very-low-density lipoprotein to LDL. The resulting large and abnormal cholesterol ester–enriched very-low-density lipoprotein is injurious to endothelial cells after receptor-mediated uptake.

Hyperglycemia appears to contribute to endothelial dysfunction as well. Hyperglycemia activates protein kinase C in endothelial cells, which in turn may account for increased production of vasoconstrictor prostaglandins, endothelia and ACE, and platelet and vascular growth factors, which directly and indirectly enhance vasomotor reactivity and vascular remodeling and growth.

Furthermore, hyperglycemia alters endothelial cell matrix production, which may contribute to basement membrane thickening. Hyperglycemia increases endothelial cell collagen IV and fibronectin synthesis and increases the activity of enzymes involved in collagen synthesis.

Hyperglycemia also delays cell replication and increases endothelial cell death in part by enhancing oxidation and glycation.

- **Diabetic Cataracts**

Dr. Obrosova et al. in the study *Diabetic cataracts: mechanisms and management*, reported that diabetes mellitus is associated with a 5-fold higher prevalence of cataracts, which remains a major cause of blindness in the world.

Typical diabetic cataracts contain cortical and/or posterior subcapsular opacities. Adult onset diabetic cataracts also often contain nuclear opacities. Both animal and human studies support important contribution of increased aldose reductase activity.

The research article *Diabetes mellitus: An overview on its pharmacological aspects and reported medicinal plants having antidiabetic activity* by Dr. Patel et al. reports that individuals with diabetes have been found to be at increased risk of visual impairment compared to non-diabetic persons.

Cataracts occur at a younger age in diabetics than non-diabetics. The incidence of cataracts increases proportionally with the degree and the period of the diabetes mellitus. It is reported that most patients having lenticular opacity had diabetes mellitus for more than five years, and that various types of opacities of the lens were developed in 64% of diabetic patients under treatment.

Caird et al. reported that 10.7% of patients with senile cataract extraction had diabetes mellitus and that the cataract extraction rate in those cases was four to six times higher than the cases without diabetes mellitus. These results indicate that the cataract incidence rate is higher in diabetes mellitus patients. In this study, the mean duration of development of cataracts in patients with diabetes mellitus was 13.03±6.96 years.

- **Prostatic Hypertrophy and Diabetes Mellitus**

Review of the pertinent medical literature shows a very clear relationship between prostatic hypertrophy and diabetes mellitus. A large study recently published, *PPARγ: A Molecular Link between systemic metabolic disease and benign prostate hyperplasia*, by Ming Jiang et al., found an excellent correlation between the size of the prostate and diabetes. The study concluded:

> "In this cohort of community-dwelling U.S. men, obesity, elevated fasting glucose, and diabetes were associated with prostate enlargement, an objective indicator of benign prostatic hyperplasia.
>
> Compared with their peers with normal range values, very obese men were 3.5-fold more likely, men with elevated glucose 3-fold more likely, and diabetic men 2-fold more likely to have an enlarged prostate.
>
> Overall obesity, rather than central obesity, appeared to be the more important predictor. The association for elevated fasting glucose in men without diabetes was attenuated, suggesting that larger perturbations in glucose homeostasis were more strongly associated with prostate enlargement.
>
> These results indicate that obesity, elevated fasting glucose, and diabetes are risk factors for benign prostatic hyperplasia and are consistent with previous observations of obesity, serum insulin, and prostate volume."

CHAPTER 11 - PSYCHIATRY

Winning a Claim for Posttraumatic Stress Disorder (PTSD) Benefits

In the past, the three main errors made by the VA in rating PTSD have been:

1. The rating officer provided a lower rating than was justified by the clinical presentation.
2. The VA concluded that the stressor the veteran experienced was not "an event that is outside the range of usual human experience and would have been markedly distressing to almost anyone."
3. There was no evidence that the veteran was actually in combat.

These conclusions by the VA are no longer acceptable reasons for denial of benefits. Recent VA rulings, Court rulings, and the replacement of the DSM-III-R with the DSM-IV and now DSM-V, as the basis for determination of disability, have dramatically changed the way the VA rates, or should rate, veterans applying for disability benefits.

The Department of Veterans' Affairs has recently published a new manual, "Best Practice Manual for Posttraumatic Stress Disorder (PTSD) Compensation and Pension Examinations.

> "With the publication of this manual, the VA has declared: "The Veterans' Benefits Administration (VBA) and Veterans' Health Administration (VHA) are committed to improving these services to veterans, and improving the quality of

compensation and pension examinations for PTSD." The manual changes many of the assumptions that led to denial of PTSD claims in the past."

Review of this manual is critical to claimants and their attorneys.

What Did the VA PTSD Study Find?

The Veterans' Benefits Administration reviewed 143 initial claims for PTSD. This study revealed that at least 8% of exams were inadequate. A common problem was that the examiner did not describe how the diagnosis met the rating listed in the manual for mental disorders, the DSM-IV.

In fact, it was noted that not only did examiners fail to list the DSM-IV criteria, but that some examiners erroneously used the DSM-III-R criteria. For example, the criterion that a veteran had experienced "an event that is outside the range of usual human experience and would have been markedly distressing to almost anyone," is a DSM-III-R criterion, not a DSM-IV criterion and is no longer acceptable.

Some other frequent errors cited in this study:

- Examiners failed to note whether other mental disorders were due in part to PTSD;

- Less than half of the examiners had the complete claim file for review;

- Examiners stated "minor PTSD symptoms" without naming them.

The study also noted reluctance by the disability rating experts and the VA to grant 100% disability; the highest rating granted was 70% despite clear indication that the veteran had severe symptoms meriting 100% disability. The authors of the study admonished: "It is no longer correct to say that total incapacitation for anxiety disorder is unusual."

In addition, it was observed that officers were often denied benefits when the Global Assessment of Functioning (GAF) Scale was 60 (i.e. moderate symptoms), while the committee requires that in cases where the GAF is 60, a 30% disability must be assigned.

Upon review of the study, the committee made the following recommendations:

- The clinician-administered PTSD scale CAPS, (Blake et al. 1995), is recommended as the interview method of choice for conducting compensation and pension examination. It requires approximately one hour, but may be abbreviated.
- Psychometric tests must never be used alone to deny rating for PTSD -- only to supplement and substantiate findings.

Professionals qualified to perform PTSD examinations should have a doctoral level training in psychopathology.

What is Posttraumatic Stress Disorder (PTSD)?

The DSM-IV has replaced the DSM-III-R, which focused solely on combat trauma. The DSM-III-R criteria required, for example, that the veteran had experienced "an event that is outside the range of human experience and would have been markedly distressing to almost anyone." This criterion is no longer acceptable under the DSM-IV.

The DSM-IV Diagnostic Criteria for PTSD:

   A. The person has been exposed to a traumatic event in which both of the following have been present:

      1. The person has experienced, witnessed or been confronted with an event or events that involve actual or threatened death or serious injury, or threat to the physical integrity of oneself or others.

      2. The person's response involved intense fear, helplessness, or horror. (They note that assault violence, particularly of a criminal nature, is more likely to induce PTSD than a random act of God. Factors surrounding the traumatic incident, such as absence of social support, may also influence the degree to which the stressful event is experienced.)

B. The traumatic event is persistently re-experienced in one or more of the following ways:

1. Recurrent and intrusive distressing recollections of the event, including images, thoughts or perceptions

2. Recurrent distressing dreams of the event

3. Acting or feeling as if the traumatic event were recurring (includes a sense of reliving the experience, illusions, hallucinations, and dissociative flashback episodes, including those that occur upon awakening or when intoxicated)

4. Intense psychological distress at exposure to internal or external cues that symbolize or resemble an aspect of the traumatic event

5. Physiological reactivity upon exposure to internal or external cues that symbolize or resemble an aspect of the traumatic event

C. Persistent avoidance of stimuli associated with the trauma

D. Persistent symptoms of increasing arousal (not present before the trauma), indicated by: difficulty in falling or staying asleep, irritability or outbursts of anger, difficulty concentrating, hyper-vigilance, exaggerated startle response

E. Duration of the disturbance (symptoms) is more than one month

F. The disturbance causes clinically significant distress or impairment in social, occupational, or other important areas of functioning.

Does a Veteran Need to Prove That He/She Was Involved in Combat for a PTSD Claim

The most common reason for denial of a well diagnosed PTSD claim, is the VA Rating Officer's conclusion that the veteran did not prove he was involved in combat. While the focus of PTSD stressors is usually combat stress, the VA now recognizes that that there are less common, but equally important stressors such as sexual harassment or sexual abuse during service.

Duties such as grave registration, morgue assignment, accidents involving injury, and even peacekeeping deployment may meet stressor criteria. What is required in a PTSD claim is that the veteran show that he/she was exposed to *a traumatic event* during his/her military service, not necessarily combat trauma.

On August 1, 2010, the Veterans' Court of Appeals in *Cohen v. Brown* 94-661 10 vet. App dramatically changed the way PTSD is evaluated and rated. The Board of Veteran Appeals denied Cohen's request for benefits, because he never served in combat. The Court reversed and held that noncombat stressors described by the veteran were sufficient to cause PTSD.

First, the Court cited that a stressor causing a veteran to suffer from PTSD need not be unusually traumatic. It is the effect of the stressor on a particular veteran that needs be assessed:

> "Under the DSM-IV, the mental illness of PTSD would be treated the same as a physical illness for purposes of VA disability compensation in terms of a predisposition toward development of that condition. For example, the court noted [that the] VA does not deny a service-connection award to a veteran whose lack of good balance causes him to fall and be injured during service even though a serviceperson with better balance would not have been injured at all."

Second, the Court held that the stressor need not be combat stress. The veteran in *Cohen v. Brown* testified that while in Vietnam he was not a combat soldier:

> "The veteran responded to the RO's inquiry by explaining that although he was assigned an MOS of power generator equipment mechanic he 'never performed these duties' and that 'most of [his] duties consisted of convoys, heavy equip[ment] mechanic [and] guard duty'. R. at 82. The military experiences he said he had considered 'most terrifying, life threatening, or stressful" included the following: (1) Armed combat or enemy action; (2) mortar and rocket attacks; (3) treating or dealing with casualties; (4) convoys; and (5) many hours of work and lack of sleep."

Finally, the Court held that the veteran's lay testimony was sufficient to establish the existence of these stressors.

Concerning the adjudication of claims for PTSD, the VBA's Adjudication Procedures Manual states:

1. PTSD does not need to have its onset during combat. For example, vehicular or airplane crashes, large fires, floods, earthquakes, and other disasters would evoke significant distress in most involved veterans. The trauma may be experienced alone (rape or assault) or in the company of groups of people (military combat).

2. A stressor is not to be limited to just one single episode. A group of experiences also may affect an individual, leading to a diagnosis of PTSD. In some circumstances, for example, assignment to a grave registration unit, burn care unit, or liberation of internment camps could have a cumulative effect of powerful, distressing experiences essential to the diagnosis of PTSD.

3. PTSD can be caused by events that occurred before, during, or after service. The relationship between stressors during military service and current problems/symptoms will govern the question of service connection. Symptoms must have a clear relationship to the military stressor as described in the medical records.

4. PTSD can occur hours, months, or years after a military stressor. Despite this long latent period, service-connected PTSD may be recognizable by a relevant association between the stressor and the current presentation of symptoms. This association between stressor and symptoms must be specifically addressed in the VA examination report and to a practical extent supported by documentation.

5. Every decision involving the issue of service connection for PTSD alleged to have occurred as a result of combat must include a factual determination as to whether or not the veteran was engaged in combat, including the reasons or bases for that finding. (See *Gaines v. West*, 11 Vet. App. 113 (1998))

A stressor is not limited to just a single episode; a group of experiences, such an assignment to a Grave Registration Unit, or a Burn Care Unit have a cumulative effect that can result in PTSD.

PTSD can be due to events, which occur before, during or after service, and not specifically in relationship to the military stressors. PTSD may present after a long latent period; even years. Thus, the rating examiner must not restrict the search for corroborating evidence of stressors to service records; other sources must be looked at as well.

In *Doran v. Brown*, 6 Vet. App. 283, 290-91 (1994), the U.S. Court of Appeals for Veterans Claims (Court) stated, "the absence of corroboration in the service records, when there is nothing in the available records that is inconsistent with other evidence, does not relieve the BVA of its obligations to assess the credibility and probative value of the other evidence." In *Doran*, the Court cited a provision of the VA ADJUDICATION PROCEDURE MANUAL M21-1 to read, in part, that "corroborating evidence of a stressor is not restricted to service records, but may be obtained from other sources."

The evidence necessary to establish the occurrence of a recognizable stressor during service - to support a diagnosis of PTSD - will vary depending upon whether the veteran engaged in "combat with the enemy," as established by recognized military combat citations or other official records. See, e.g., *Hayes v. Brown*, 5 Vet. App. 60, 66 (1993); *Doran v. Brown*, 6 Vet. App. 283, 289 (1994).

When there is a current diagnosis of PTSD, the sufficiency of the claimed in-service stressor is presumed. *Cohen*, 10 Vet. App. at 144. Nevertheless, credible evidence that the claimed in-service stressor actually occurred is still required. 38 C.F.R. § 3.304(f). And credible supporting evidence of the actual occurrence of an in-service stressor cannot consist solely of after-the-fact medical nexus evidence. See *Moreau v. Brown*, 9 Vet. App. 389, 396 (1996). Corroboration does not require, however, "that there be corroboration of every detail including the appellant's personal participation in the identifying process." *Suozzi v. Brown*, 10 Vet. App. 307, 311 (1997).

What Evidence is Required to Prove Combat Stressors?

The following conclusive evidence is sufficient to prove combat stressors:

> "Any evidence available from the service department indicating that the veteran served in the area in which the stressful event is alleged to have occurred and any evidence supporting the description of the event are to be made part of the record. Corroborating evidence of a stressor is not restricted to service records, but may be obtained from other sources (see *Doran v. Brown*, 6 Vet. App. 283 (1994)). If the claimed stressor is related to combat, in the absence of information to the contrary, receipt of any of the following individual decorations will be considered evidence of participation in a stressful episode:
>
> - Air Force Cross
> - Air Medal with "V" Device
> - Army Commendation Medal with "V" Device
> - Bronze Star Medal with "V" Device
> - Combat Action Ribbon
> - Combat Infantryman Badge
> - Combat Medical Badge
> - Distinguished Flying Cross
> - Distinguished Service Cross
> - Joint Service Commendation Medal with "V" Device
> - Medal of Honor

- Navy Commendation Medal with "V" Device
- Navy Cross
- Purple Heart
- Silver Star

Other supportive evidence includes, but is not limited to: plane crash, ship sinking, explosion, rape or assault, duty in a burn ward or in a grave registration unit. POW status, which satisfies the requirements of 38 CFR 3.1(y), will also be considered conclusive evidence of an in-service stressor."

Mere presence in a combat zone is not sufficient to show that a veteran actually engaged in combat with enemy forces. *Wood v. Derwinski*, 1 Vet. App. 190, 193 (1991), affirmed on reconsideration, 1 Vet. App. 406 (1991). On the other hand, whether a veteran has submitted sufficient corroborative evidence of claimed in-service stressors is a factual determination. *Pentecost v. Principi*, 16 Vet. App. 124 (2002).

And in both *Pentecost* and *Suozzi*, it was held that specific evidence that a veteran was actually with his unit at the time of an attack is not required to verify that attack as a PTSD stressor. *Pentecost*, 16 Vet. App. at 128 (holding that the Board erred in "insisting that there be corroboration of the veteran's personal participation"); *Suozzi*, 10 Vet. App. 310-11 (evidence that veteran's company received heavy casualties during an attack, even without specific evidence that the veteran was "integrally involved in the attack" was sufficient to reopen his claim for service connection for PTSD).

Pursuant to the holdings in *Pentecost* and *Suozzi*, there does not need to be corroboration of each and every detail of a veteran's personal participation in the alleged combat activity in Vietnam. Rather, the mere fact that his unit was involved in that combat activity is reason enough, alone, to presume that he experienced the type of stressor alleged in that capacity. Thus, his combat stressor must be conceded, particularly when all reasonable doubt is resolved in his favor concerning this. See 38 C.F.R. § 3.102; *Alemany v. Brown*, 9 Vet. App. 518, 519 (1996).

What Evidence is Required to Prove a Personal or Sexual Assault?

Cases involving PTSD as a result of a personal or sexual assault pose a particular problem. Evidence of personal assault may be lacking. The examiner must look at other supporting documents that may prove the existence of a stressor; a visit to a medical or counseling clinic without a specific diagnosis, or a specific ailment, or a sudden request for transfer, may suggest the existence of a sexual assault.

Lay statement regarding leave without absence, change in performance, episode of depression by lay statement, increased or decreased use of prescription medication or over-the-counter medication, evidence of substance abuse such as alcohol, and unexplained economic or social behavior changes, may all point to the occurrence of a specific traumatic experience.

Personal assault is an event of human design that threatens or inflicts harm. Examples of personal assault are rape, physical assault, domestic battery, robbery, mugging, and stalking. If the military record contains no documentation that a personal assault occurred, alternative evidence might still establish an in-service stressful incident. Behavior changes that occurred at the time of the incident may indicate the occurrence of an in-service stressor.

Examples of behavior changes that may indicate a stressor include (but are not limited to):

- Visits to a medical or counseling clinic or dispensary without a specific diagnosis or specific ailment
- Sudden requests that the veteran's military occupational series or duty assignment be changed without other justification
- Lay statements indicating increased use or abuse of leave without any apparent reason such as family obligations or family illness
- Changes in performance and performance evaluations
- Lay statements describing episodes of depression, panic attacks, or anxiety, but no identifiable reasons for the episodes
- Increased or decreased use of prescription medications
- Increased use of over-the-counter medications

- Evidence of substance abuse such as alcohol or drugs
- Increased disregard for military or civilian authority
- Obsessive behavior such as overeating or under eating
- Pregnancy tests around the time of the incident
- Increased interest in tests for HIV or sexually transmitted diseases
- Unexplained economic or social behavior changes
- Treatment for physical injuries around the time of the claimed trauma, but not reported as a result of the trauma
- Breakup of a primary relationship

In personal assault claims, secondary evidence may need interpretation by a clinician, especially if it involves behavior changes. Evidence that documents such behavior changes may require interpretation in relationship to the medical diagnosis by a VA neuropsychiatric physician.

Is the Veteran's Own Testimony Sufficient to Establish a Stressor?

A combat veteran's lay testimony alone may establish an in-service stressor for purposes of service connecting PTSD (*Cohen v. Brown*, 94-661 (U.S. Ct. Vet. App. March 7, 1997)). However, a noncombat veteran's testimony alone does not qualify as "credible supporting evidence" of the occurrence of an in-service stressor as required by 38 CFR 3.304(f). After-the-fact psychiatric analyses which infer a traumatic event are likewise insufficient in this regard (*Moreau v. Brown*, 9 Vet. App. 389 (1996)).

Alcohol and Drug Abuse in PTSD Cases

The VA is prohibited by statute, 38 U.S.C. § 1110, from paying compensation to a veteran whose disability is a result of his own alcohol and drug abuse. However, when a veteran's alcohol or drug abuse disability is secondary to or is a result of or aggravated by a primary service-connected disorder, the veteran may be entitled to compensation. See *Allen v. Principi*, 237 F.3d 1368, 1381 (Fed. Cir. 2001).

Therefore, it is important to determine the relationship, if any, between a service-connected disorder and a disability resulting from the veteran's alcohol or drug abuse. The rating officer should separate, to the extent possible, the effects of the alcohol or drug abuse from the effects of the other mental disorder(s). If it is not possible to separate the effects in such cases, an explanation must be given.

In *Allen v. Principi*, 237 F.3d 1368 (Fed. Cir., 2001) the Court held:

> "We therefore conclude, based on the language of the statute and the pertinent legislative history, that 38 U.S.C. § 1110 does not preclude compensation for an alcohol or drug abuse

disability secondary to a service-connected disability or use of an alcohol or drug abuse disability as evidence of the increased severity of a service-connected disability. We would stress that the holding of the case is quite limited. Veterans can only recover if they can adequately establish that their alcohol or drug abuse disability is secondary to or is caused by their primary service- connected disorder. We foresee that such compensation would only result where there is clear medical evidence establishing that the alcohol or drug abuse disability is indeed caused by a veteran's primary service-connected disability, and where the alcohol or drug abuse disability is not due to willful wrongdoing.

On remand, the Board will have to determine whether Allen's alcohol abuse disability is secondary to his PTSD, or whether it demonstrates the increased severity of his PTSD disability. If it finds sufficient evidence demonstrating a causal connection, Allen could be entitled to an increase in his schedular rating. But if the Board finds that Allen's alcohol abuse is willful and did not result from his PTSD, Allen could not receive additional compensation for a willful alcohol abuse disability."

Psychological Testing in PTSD Claims

Regarding psychological testing, the Committee recommended the use of the Minnesota Multiphasic Personality Inventory (MMPI). The Committee did caution that inherent in the test is the risk of over-reporting, citing validity scales that are elevated in people who attempt to exaggerate their symptoms. However, studies of Vietnam combat veterans and child abuse survivors show elevated scores as a result of chronic posttraumatic difficulties or comorbid affective symptoms as opposed to over endorsement.

In 1997, the Veterans' Administration mandated that a GAF (Global Assessment of Functioning) score be assigned at regular intervals for veterans receiving mental health care. The GAF score is often used in disability rating boards and was included in the DSM profile.
A high GAF may be erroneously assigned to a Veteran suffering from PTSD because his symptom severity and functionality can fluctuate. Studies have also shown that the difference in GAF scores assigned by different raters for the same patient could easily vary by 20 points; where one rater considered the symptoms to be mild and the other judged them to be moderate to severe, and it is often seen that raters vary by as much as 8 points on the same examination. The Committee also noted that Veterans' Administration practitioners seem to have a bias against assigning low GAF scores for PTSD; thus, a high GAF (>61) by itself, should not be a reason to deny veteran disability benefits.

In addition, there is no published information associated with the DSM-IV, which instructs examiners on the valid methods for partitioning the GAF score by comorbid clinical condition. It is VBA policy that the examiner must assign GAF scores for comorbid disorders. If he does not do so, he is required to explain why. Failure to address comorbid mental conditions, such as depression or anxiety, has been seen as a major error in rating decisions that must be corrected.

The Committee stressed the importance of recording episodes of aggression against self or others. If applied correctly, these behaviors will drop the GAF into a lower range. If these features are present clinically, they should not be overlooked or minimized by the clinician.

Finally, the Committee recommended that the GAF score should only be used as a crosscheck against the examiner's own evaluation, based on reports of signs and symptoms; if they do not match, the practitioner is advised to re-examine the evidence. However, there is no reason to change an evaluation because the GAF score differs in the assessment level of functioning from that of the evaluation

Rating Considerations for PTSD

A Veteran is Entitled to a PTSD Disability Rating of 70% due to a GAF of 45 and the Inability to Work

In *Johnson v. Brown*, 7 Vet. App. 95 (1994), the Court determined the criteria for granting benefits for a mental disorder described under a 70% rating (as well as ratings of 100%, 50% and 30%). The criteria focus on: (1) a veteran's ability to "maintain effective or favorable relationships with people" and, (2) the effect of the psychoneurotic symptoms on the veteran's ability "to obtain or retain employment." The Court also held that the two criteria for a 70% rating under 38 C.F.R. §

4.132, DC 9411 (1996) are each independent of the other.

The Global Assessment of Functioning (GAF) scale reflects the psychological, social, and occupational functioning under a hypothetical continuum of mental illness. See American Psychiatric Association's Diagnostic and Statistical Manual of Mental Disorders (4th ed. 1994) (DSM-IV); see also *Carpenter v. Brown*, 8 Vet. App. 240, 243 (1995):

> "A GAF score between 41 and 50 is indicative of serious symptoms (e.g., suicidal ideation, severe obsessional rituals, frequent shoplifting) or any serious impairment in social, occupational, or school functioning (e.g. no friends, unable to keep a job). Id.
>
> A GAF score between 51 and 60 is indicative of moderate symptoms (e.g., flat affect and circumstantial speech, occasional panic attacks) or moderate difficulty in social, occupational, or school functioning (e.g., few friends, conflicts with peers or coworkers). Id."

The Board explained how the GAF score is used in a rating decision, Citation Nr: 0304543, Decision Date: 03/12/03, DOCKET NO. 96-45 560A:

> "A 70% disability rating is assigned when the ability to establish and maintain effective or favorable relationships with people is severely impaired. The psychoneurotic symptoms are of

such severity and persistence that there is severe impairment in the ability to obtain or retain employment.

A 50% disability rating is assigned when the ability to establish or maintain effective and wholesome relationships with people is considerably impaired. By reason of psychoneurotic symptoms, the reliability, flexibility and efficiency levels are so reduced as to result in considerable industrial impairment."

The Court has held that if any one of the three independent criteria contained in Diagnostic Code 9411 in effect prior to November 7, 1996, is met, a 100 schedular evaluation is required under that code. *Johnson v. Brown*, 7 Vet. App. 95, 99 (1994).

When the only compensable service-connected disability is a mental disability, and such mental disorder precludes a veteran from securing or following a substantially gainful occupation, the mental disorder shall be assigned a 100% schedular evaluation under the appropriate diagnostic code. 38 C.F.R. § 4.16 (c) (1996).

When there is a question as to which of two evaluations shall be assigned, the higher evaluation will be assigned if the disability picture more nearly approximates the criteria for that rating. Otherwise, the lower rating will be assigned. 38 C.F.R. § 4.7.

According to the Diagnostic and Statistical Manual of Mental Disorders, Fourth Edition (DSM-IV), a GAF score of between 51 and 60 means that the veteran has moderate symptoms (flat affect and circumstantial speech, occasional panic attacks) OR moderate difficulty in social, occupational, or school functioning (e.g., few friends, conflicts with peers or co-workers). A GAF score of between 41 and 50 means that the veteran has either serious symptoms or serious difficulty in social, occupational, or school functioning.

In *Mittleider v. West*, 11 Vet. App. 181, 182 (1998), the Court quoted a passage from the Federal Register indicating that when it is not possible to separate the effects of a service-connected condition from non-service-connected conditions, "VA regulations at 38 C.F.R. § 3.102 . . . clearly dictate that such signs and symptoms be attributed to the service-connected condition." See also Citation Nr: 1331147, Decision Date: 09/27/13, Archive Date: 10/01/13, DOCKET NO. 08-22 151.

In *Bowling v. Principi*, No. 99-2264 (2001), the Court acknowledged that a GAF score of 50 represents "serious" impairment:

> "The Board cited this Court's opinion in *Carpenter (Eugene) v. Brown*, 8 Vet.App. 240, 242 (1995). However, in that case where there was no evidence of a GAF score below 55, the Court held that where a veteran has "had a GAF of 55 to 60" that score "corresponds to 'moderate difficulty in social, occupational, or school

functioning'", ibid. (emphasis added) (quoting Diagnostic and Statistical Manual of Mental Disorders 32 (4th ed. 1994) [hereinafter DSM-IV]), and that the veteran was thus not entitled to a 70% rating under DC 9411. In contrast, in the instant case, the veteran's GAF score has been recorded as being as low as 45 ... *Cf. Richard (Mary) v. Brown*, 9 Vet.App. 266 (1996) (veteran with PTSD rated at 70% received GAF score of 50). In *Richard (Mary)*, the Court recognized that a GAF score of 50 indicated "'serious'" impairment. Id. at 267-68 (emphasis added) (quoting DSM-IV at 32). On remand, the Board must explain why in this case, where the most recent evidence showed GAF scores of 50 twice in January 1999 and 53 in the prior year (R. at 700, 706) and where other recent evidence showed a GAF score of 50 (R. at 691), the Board chose to characterize the veteran's GAF score range as "55-60" and thereby apply *Carpenter (Eugene)*, rather than to characterize the veteran's GAF score range as, for example, "50-53", and consider the veteran to have either "serious" symptoms or "serious" impairment as described in the DSM-IV criteria discussed in *Richard (Mary) v. Brown*."

Hypertension Secondary to PTSD

There is a relationship between PTSD and the development of hypertension. It is now abundantly clear that PTSD is associated with aberrations of rapid eye movement sleep resulting in the development of hypertension.

Individuals with PTSD often report sleep disturbances including trouble in falling and maintaining sleep, recurrent nightmares about trauma, and other disruptive nocturnal behaviors such as anxiety and night terrors during sleep.

Veterans with PTSD have a higher prevalence of obstructive sleep apnea (OSA) than the general population. Untreated OSA accentuates the sleep-related symptoms of PTSD, especially the number and intensity of nightmares, repeated awakenings, difficulty falling back to sleep, and increase in daytime sleepiness and tiredness.

A growing body of evidence suggests that disturbed sleep is more likely to be a core feature of PTSD rather than just a secondary symptom. Hypoxia, sympathetic discharge from respiratory disturbances, dysfunctional REM sleep, and abnormal REM mechanism have been proposed as mechanisms for sleep apnea in PTSD patients.

Kobayashi et al. conducted a meta-analytic review of 20 polysomnographic studies comparing sleep in people with and without PTSD. Results showed that PTSD patients had more stage 1 sleep, less slow wave sleep, and greater rapid-eye-movement density compared to people without PTSD.

A recent study showed that treatment of OSA with CPAP is associated with a decrease in the number of nightmares and daytime sleepiness in PTSD patients.

This study also showed a positive correlation of REM sleep percentage with the number of nightmares. This supports the hypothesis that dysfunctional REM sleep mechanism may be involved in the pathogenesis of PTSD. A recent study reported that REM AHI and interrupted sleep at night were independent predictors of nightmares in OSA patients, and CPAP therapy results in significant improvement in nightmare occurrence. Apparently when a patient spends more time in REM the likelihood of having nightmares becomes higher. REM suppression with prazosin, an α-1 inhibitor, showed improvement in combat-related PTSD nightmares and sleep quality in active-duty soldiers in a recent trial. This may indicate that suppressing the "dysfunctional REM" in PTSD patients may have helped reduce symptoms.

Taken together, these studies show that patients suffering from PTSD have abnormalities of their REM sleep which is associated with development of nightmares. Treatment by CPAP not only ameliorates sleep apnea symptoms but also improves PTSD symptoms.

Rapid-eye-movement sleep (REM sleep) physiologically entails arterial pressure surges. Pressure surges may lead to acute cardiovascular events in risk conditions such as arterial hypertension. REM sleep is a state of heightened vegetative variability, the manifestations of which, in healthy human subjects include phasic increases (surges) of arterial pressure. In physiologic conditions, pressure surges have also been described during REM sleep in animal models, thus being a remarkably robust feature of this sleep state.

Although pressure surges may result from an enhancement of cardiovascular variability in different behavioral conditions, their characteristics appear of substantial interest during REM sleep. The pressure surges in REM sleep critically depend on central neural mechanisms, which may be intrinsic to the brain processes of this state.

Moreover, it has been hypothesized that the pressure surges during REM sleep in the last part of the night contribute to the increased incidence of acute cardiovascular events, which is observed in the early morning hours after awakening. In fact, pressure surges may induce atherosclerotic plaque rupture and thrombosis, representing an acute risk factor for myocardial infarction, sudden cardiac death, and stroke.

The VA itself has recognized a link between hypertension and PTSD; specifically, when the VA established hypertensive vascular disease as a disease presumptively related to the prisoner of war ("POW") experience. The VA relied on several studies finding that PTSD was a risk factor for hypertension. See Presumptions of Service Connection for Diseases Associated With Service Involving Detention or Internment as a Prisoner of War, 69 Fed. Reg, 60,083,60,087 (Oct. 1, 2004) (Interim Final Rule amending 38 C.F.R. § 3.309(c)). For example, the agency cited a 2003 VA study that found a "statistically significant increased incidence of hypertension and chronic heart disease among World War II veterans with PTSD..." The VA also cited a 1997 study finding that Vietnam veterans diagnosed with PTSD had a significantly increased risk of circulatory disease many years after service."

CHAPTER 12 - TOXICOLOGY

Agent Orange

Concerns about the toxicity of Agent Orange and its health effects led the U.S. Department of Veterans' Affairs and The Institute of Medicine of the U.S. National Academy of Sciences (IOM) to conduct a biennial and cumulative epidemiological review of herbicide exposure. The evidence is not based on causality but on the strength of epidemiological evidence associating herbicide exposure with health.

The IOM report classifies the evidence in support of a relationship as 'sufficient', 'limited or suggestive', or 'inadequate or insufficient'. The cancers included in the 'sufficient evidence' list in the 2010 update are soft-tissue sarcoma (including heart); non-Hodgkin lymphoma (NHL); chronic lymphocytic leukemia (CLL) (including hairy cell leukemia and other chronic B-cell leukemias) and Hodgkin disease. Those on the 'limited or suggestive' list are laryngeal cancer; cancer of the lung, bronchus or trachea; prostate cancer and multiple myeloma.

In a report to the Secretary of the Department of Veterans' Affairs on the association between adverse health effects and exposure to Agent Orange dated May 5, 1990, Admiral E.R. Zumwalt, Jr. stated:

> "On October 6, 1989 I was appointed as special assistant to Secretary Derwinski of the Department of Veterans Affairs to assist the Secretary in determining whether it is at least as

likely as not that there is a statistical association between exposure to Agent Orange and a specific adverse health effect.

After reviewing the scientific literature related to the health effects of Vietnam Veterans exposed to Agent Orange as well as other studies concerning the health hazards of civilian exposure to dioxin contaminants, I conclude that there is adequate evidence for the Secretary to reasonably conclude that it is at least as likely as not that there is a relationship between exposure to Agent Orange and the following health problems: non—Hodgkin's lymphoma, chloracne and other skin disorders, lip cancer, bone cancer, soft tissue sarcoma, birth defects, skin cancer, porphyria cutanea tarda and other liver disorders, Hodgkin's disease, hematopoietic diseases, multiple myeloma, neurological defects, auto—immune diseases and disorders, leukemia, lung cancer, kidney cancer, malignant melanoma, pancreatic cancer, stomach cancer, colon cancer, nasal/pharyngeal/esophageal cancers, prostate cancer, testicular cancer, liver cancer, brain cancer, psychosocial effects and gastrointestinal diseases."

UNITED STATES COURT OF APPEALS FOR VETERANS CLAIMS No. 06-3024
DEANNA R. POLOVICK, APPELLANT, V. ERIC K. SHINSEKI

Title 38, section 1116(b)(1) of the U.S. Code directs the Secretary to "prescribe regulations providing that a presumption of service connection is warranted for [a] disease" when a positive statistical association exists between Agent Orange exposure and the occurrence of that disease in humans.

The statute further provides that a positive association exists when "the credible evidence for the association is equal to or outweighs the credible evidence against the association." In making this determination the Secretary is to take into account reports from the National Academy of Sciences under section 3 of the Agent Orange Act of 1991 as well as all other available sound medical and scientific information. 38 U.S.C. § 1116(b)(3).

To carry out this directive, the National Academy of Sciences convened an IOM committee to answer, whether a statistical association with herbicide exposure exists. Even though a disease is not included on the list of presumptive diseases, a nexus between the disease and service may nevertheless be established on the basis of direct service connection. See *Stefl v. Nicholson*, 21 Vet. App. 120, 123 (2007) ("The existence of presumptive service connection for a condition based on exposure to Agent Orange presupposes that it is possible for medical evidence to prove such a link before the National Academy of Sciences recognizes a positive association."). Of particular relevance to an analysis of medical evidence supporting such a nexus are factors such as whether a medical professional finds studies persuasive,

UNITED STATES COURT OF APPEALS FOR VETERANS CLAIMS NO. 04-2192
BARNEY J. STEFL, APPELLANT, V. R. JAMES NICHOLSON

"[T]he physician mistakenly assumed that, since the appellant's nasal sinus disease was not included in the list of presumptive service-connected diseases, it could not be related to service."

A medical nexus opinion finding a condition is not related to service *because* the condition is not entitled to presumptive service connection, without clearly considering direct service connection, is inadequate on its face. Without a medical opinion that clearly addresses the relevant facts and medical science, the Board is left to rely on its own lay opinion, which it is forbidden from doing. *See Colvin v. Derwinski*, 1 Vet. App. 171, 175 (1991) (holding that the Board may only consider independent medical evidence and may not substitute its own medical opinion.)

Oral Cancer Caused by Exposure to Agent Orange

The IOM noted that oral cancer could be lumped into a broader category of respiratory cancers including cancer of the larynx and the bronchus. It is a logical conclusion as Agent Orange was inhaled by the soldiers who were exposed to it, and thus, had great exposure to the agent in the oral cavity, larynx and bronchus.

> "Oral, nasal, and pharyngeal cancers are found in many anatomic subsites, including the structures of the mouth (inside lining of the lips, cheeks, gums, tongue, and hard and soft palate) (ICD-9 140-145), oropharynx (ICD-9 146), nasopharynx (ICD-9 147), hypopharynx (ICD-9 148), other buccal cavity and pharynx (ICD-9 149), and nasal cavity and paranasal sinuses (ICD-9 160). Although those sites are anatomically diverse, cancers that occur in the nasal cavity, oral cavity, and pharynx are for the most part similar in descriptive epidemiology and risk factors. The exception is cancer of the nasopharynx, which has a different epidemiologic profile."

The BVA determined that the veteran's oral cancer was caused by Agent Orange because he did not have risk factors normally linked to oral cancer and because the cancer is similar to the cancer of the larynx and trachea which are already presumed by the VA to because of exposure to the herbicide:

> "The opinions offered by the veteran's treating oncologist- who is affiliated with the Kansas City VA Medical Center in Kansas City, Missouri- support the veteran's claim that his exposure to Agent Orange contributed to his cancer. In these letters, the oncologist linked the veteran's mouth cancer to his exposure to Agent Orange and noted specifically that the veteran had no other risk factors for the disease, to include heavy drinking, smoking, or other use of tobacco products. In fact, the oncologist stated in his January 2007 letter that the likelihood that the veteran's mouth

cancer 'was caused by Agent Orange is as great, if not greater, than anyone who has been service-connected for any respiratory disorder. There is absolutely no speculation in this regard.' Similarly, the treating oncologist stated in a November 2005 letter that he found it 'extremely likely that Agent Orange contributed to the development" of the veteran's mouth cancer. Additionally, a second VA oncologist supplied an opinion in August 2006 concluding that the veteran's mouth cancer could be rationally linked to Agent Orange exposure, particularly in light of the fact that other aerodigestive cancers, such as cancer of the larynx and trachea, are already presumed by VA to be caused by exposure to the herbicide. Significantly, the Board notes that there is no medical evidence in the record to suggest that the veteran's mouth cancer is not caused by his in-service exposure to Agent Orange."

The research article, *The mortality and cancer experience of New Zealand Vietnam war veterans: a cohort study*, by Dr. David McBride et al. reports that between 1964 and 1975 nearly 3400 New Zealand military personnel served in the Republic of Vietnam. There were 159 (39.1%) 'all cancer' deaths with a significantly higher SMR for cancers of the head and neck (SMR 2.20, 95% CI 1.09 to 3.93), in particular cancers of the oral cavity, pharynx and larynx (SMR 2.13, 95% CI 1.06 to 3.81).

Cause of death	Observed	Expected	SMR	95% CI*
Prostate cancer	13	12.6	1.03	0.55 to 1.76
Lung cancer	50	43.6	1.15	0.85 to 1.51
Head and neck*	11	5.0	2.20	1.09 to 3.93
Oral cavity, pharynx and larynx†	11	5.2	2.13	1.06 to 3.81
Larynx	2	1.0	2.00	0.23 to 7.39

Cause of death	Observed	Expected	SMR	95% CI*
Hodgkin disease	1	0.4	2.30	0.03 to 12.8

In reviewing the data from this study, it is abundantly clear that oral cavity cancer was actually more prevalent in soldiers who served in Vietnam than soldiers who died from prostate cancer and Hodgkin disease, two cancers that are now clearly recognized by the Veterans' Administration as presumptive Agent Orange caused cancers.

Myelodysplastic Syndrome (MDS) Due to Exposure to Agent Orange

The Myelodysplastic Syndromes (MDS) comprise a group of malignant blood stem cell disorders characterized by dysplastic and ineffective blood cell production and a risk of transformation to acute leukemia. 25-35% of patients with MDS progress to leukemia.

There is strong scientific data that links exposure to Agent Orange to the development of MDS. Patients with MDS suffer from a reduction in the production of normal red blood cells, platelets, and mature granulocytes. This often results in a variety of systemic consequences including anemia, bleeding, and an increased risk of infection.

Reports from the American Cancer Society clearly show that a third of the patients suffering from MDS will develop an acute myeloid leukemia. The American Cancer Society reports:

> "Myelodysplastic syndromes (MDS) are conditions that occur when the blood-forming cells in the bone marrow are damaged. This damage leads to low numbers of one or more types of blood cells. MDS is considered a type of cancer...
>
> In MDS, some of the cells in the bone marrow are damaged and have problems making new blood cells. Many of the blood cells formed by the damaged bone marrow cells are defective. Defective cells often die earlier than normal cells and the body also destroys some abnormal blood cells, leaving the patient with low blood counts because there aren't enough normal blood cells...
>
> In about one-third of patients, MDS can progress to a rapidly growing cancer of bone marrow cells called acute myeloid leukemia."

There is additional strong evidence to show that MDS is a known precursor to Non-Hodgkin's Lymphoma. Numerous scholarly sources support this contention.

The Board of Veterans' Appeals (Decision date April 17, 2008, Citation Nr: 0812788, Docket No. 03-11 902A) has granted service connection for myelodysplastic syndrome (MDS) claimed to be as a result of dioxin or benzene exposure in service. The case came before the Board on appeal from a May 2002 rating decision. In May 2005, the Board denied entitlement to the disability claimed and the veteran took his appeal to the United States Court of Appeals for Veterans Claims (Court). Pursuant to a joint motion the Court returned the case to the Board, which then requested a written opinion from a medical expert which follows:

> "The chemical structure of Agent Orange is composed of Benzene Rings, and it is as likely as not that exposure to Agent Orange also involves exposure to the effects of its components, that is Benzene constituents. Benzene is a known causative agent of acute myeloid leukemia, and is extensively documented in medical and environmental literature. A specific report summary by the Institute of Medicine, Gulf War and Health: A Literature Review of Pesticides and Solvents (2003) determined that there was sufficient evidence of causal relationship of Benzene to Acute Leukemia was well other bone marrow damage (Aplastic Anemia). Other articles for Benzene induced leukemia have appeared in recent peer reviewed journals. I have also reviewed the previous evaluation letter in this dispute by (M.D.B., M.D.) and agree with his reasoning and conclusion. Having reviewed all records submitted in this case, I believe the preponderance of the evidence of exposure to dibenzo-p-dioxins (Agent Orange and solvents)

and the association with the veteran's Myelodysplasia/Leukemia should be resolved in the veteran's favor. It is at least as likely as not that there is a relationship/ association/causative effect between the exposure to the pesticide/solvents used in its distribution and his MDS/Leukemia as described by medical literature in both animal and human exposures."

Hypertension, Vascular Disease and Chronic Respiratory Diseases Due to Exposure to Agent Orange

U.S. Army Chemical Corps veterans handled and sprayed herbicides in Vietnam resulting in exposure to Agent Orange and its contaminant 2,3,7, 8-tetrachlorodibenzo-p-dioxin (TCDD or dioxin). A report by Han K. Kang et al. from the Veterans Health Administration, Department of Veterans Affairs, Washington, and National Center for Environmental Health, Centers for Disease Control and Prevention, Atlanta, Georgia in *Am. J. Ind. Med.* 49:875 — 884, 2006 observed statistically significant associations between a reported history of spraying herbicide while in the military and the self-reported history of physician- diagnosed diabetes, heart disease, hypertension, and chronic respiratory diseases among this cohort of Army Chemical Corps personnel.

The positive finding of an association between phenoxy-herbicide exposure and circulatory diseases (including hypertension requiring medication) is also consistent with the results reported in other occupational/community cohorts.

An association between dioxin exposure and the risk of non-malignant lung diseases has been reported. In the 15-year period after the Seveso accident, increased deaths from chronic obstructive pulmonary disease (RR — 3.7, 95% CI — 1.4-9.9) were found in the male residents of the area where dioxin contamination was the highest (Zone A) [Pesatori et al., 1998]. Reporting of poor health and functional limitation by herbicide sprayers is consistent with an observation among the 158 BASF chemical plant workers accidentally exposed to dioxin in 1953. Their overall illness rates were positively correlated with serum dioxin concentrations and the increased illness rates were observed throughout the 36-year period and not just in the early years after the exposure [Zober et al., 1994].

In summary, almost three decades after Vietnam service, U.S. Army veterans who were occupationally exposed to phenoxyherbicide in Vietnam experienced significantly higher risks of diabetes, heart disease, hypertension, and non-malignant lung diseases than other veterans who were not exposed to herbicides.

Bladder Cancer Due to Exposure to Agent Orange

In the latest update by the Institute of Medicine Veterans and Agent Orange: Update 2014, The committee reported that Bladder cancer and hypothyroidism were moved to the "limited or suggestive" category from their previous positions in the default "inadequate or insufficient" category;

findings from the reports on the cohort of Korean veterans who served in Vietnam provided the impetus for the committee to scrutinize the previously assembled evidence on these two conditions:

> "The committee notes the consistency of these findings with the biologic understanding of the clonal derivation of lymphohematopoietic cancers that is the basis of the World Health Organization classification system (Campo et al., 2011; indicated high potential for herbicide exposure as compared to those with low potential for exposure. Among the previously reviewed epidemiology studies concerning bladder cancer and exposure to the chemicals of interest, the most comprehensive pooled analyses of workers who produced dioxin-contaminated phenoxy herbicides was published by IARC in 1997. It reported a modest increase in mortality from bladder cancer that was not extreme enough to be considered significant by usual statistical standards. The committee noted, however, a distinct pattern of elevated mortality from bladder cancer among worker groups updated for mortality after their earlier findings were incorporated in the IARC analysis. Considering that bladder cancer is predominantly a cancer of old age, it is plausible that such suggestive findings would only become apparent as the cohorts became older."

During the Vietnam War, between 1961 and 1971, the U.S. and allied forces sprayed herbicides for military purposes. The herbicides, containing phenoxy herbicides as a major ingredient, were coded as Agent Green, Orange, Pink, Purple, and White. During the manufacturing process, 2,4,5-T, an ingredient of phenoxy herbicides, was contaminated by 2,3,7,8-tetrachlorodibenzo-p-dioxin (TCDD), the most toxic dioxin congener. The TCDD being used during the Vietnam War surpassed 1000 times the permitted density limits. It is estimated that the total amount of dioxin sprayed during the Vietnam War ranged from the minimum of 366 kg to the maximum of 1000 kg.

From the initial deployment of a support unit in 1964 until its complete withdrawal in 1973, the Korean military sent 320,000 military personnel. It is presumed that many Korean Vietnam veterans were exposed to toxic herbicides, including TCDD. TCDD is being classified by the International Agency for Research on Cancer (IARC) as a group 1 carcinogen that is carcinogenic to humans. Likewise, the US National Toxicology Program listed it as a known human carcinogen.

Sang-Wook Yi et al. have shown that the 320,000 Korean Veterans who served in Vietnam compared to the general population, had a significantly elevated incidence of prostate cancer, and a marginally significantly elevated incidence of T-cell lymphoma (C84), a type of non-Hodgkin lymphoma. Overall, the Korean Vietnam veterans and military rank subcohorts had higher incidences of several cancers, including prostate cancer, T-cell lymphoma, lung cancer, bladder cancer, kidney cancer, and colon cancer than those of the general population. Prostate cancer, non-Hodgkin lymphoma, and lung cancer have been shown to have relationships with TCDD or military herbicides in a previous literature review. Several studies on the IARC phenoxy herbicide cohort, National Institute for Occupational Safety and Health cohort, and Ranch hand veterans, who were occupationally exposed to high levels of TCDD, have reported that the mortality from urinary system cancer, including bladder cancer and kidney cancer, was higher in TCDD-exposed workers and veterans than in control groups.

Prostate Cancer and Trichloroethylene (TCE) Exposure

The occurrence of prostate cancer in young individuals is an extremely rare event. The National Cancer Institute, Surveillance, Epidemiology and End Results (SEER) Program reports first time detection of prostate cancer at age under 60 is 2.3%.

A large body of epidemiologic evidence exists for exploring causal associations between cancer and trichloroethylene (TCE) exposure. The U.S. Environmental Protection Agency 2001 draft TCE health risk assessment concluded that epidemiologic studies, overall, support associations between TCE exposure and excess risk of kidney cancer, liver cancer, lymphomas, cervical cancer and prostate cancer.

The U.S. EPA draft TCE assessment noted that epidemiologic studies, when considered as a whole, have associated TCE exposure with excess risk of kidney, liver, lymphohematopoietic, cervical, and prostate cancer. Recently published studies appear to provide further support for several of those conclusions, suggesting, as do previous studies, modestly elevated site-specific risk (typically between 1.5 and 2.0), given exposure conditions in the epidemiologic studies.

The epidemiologic analysis in the U.S. EPA draft TCE risk assessment was supported in large part by the review by Wartenberg et al. (2000). This review identified more than 80 studies that evaluated cancer and TCE exposure, concluding that the evidence more firmly supported associations of TCE exposure with kidney and liver cancer while providing some support for associations with non-Hodgkin lymphoma (NHL). Wartenberg et al. (2000) also noted possible associations between TCE exposure and multiple myeloma and prostate, laryngeal, and colon cancer as well as cervical cancer and TCE or perchloroethylene exposure.

The authors compiled a list of chemicals reported to the TURA program (1990 to 2010) for which research evidence demonstrates suggestive links with prostate cancer. All chemicals are considered known human carcinogens by at least one authoritative institution. Evidence supporting the classification of these chemicals as known carcinogens comes from studies examining links between exposure and cancer types other than prostate cancer.

The association between exposure to metalworking fluids/mineral oils and increased risk of prostate cancer was further examined in a study of workers in the auto industry. This study demonstrated modest elevations of prostate cancer risk with increasing cumulative exposure to soluble and straight mineral oils that occurred 5 years or more before diagnosis.

The exposure-response relationship with soluble fluids was determined as non-linear with significantly increased risk occurring at the highest exposure level of 270 mg/m^3-years (RR=3.41). In contrast the exposure-response relationship between prostate cancer and straight fluids was linear resulting in a significant 12% increase in risk for every increase of 10 mg/m^3-years of cumulative exposure.

In a second study using data from this same cohort of auto-industry workers, risk of prostate cancer increased linearly with exposure to metalworking fluids from puberty to early adulthood (RR=2.4 per 10 mg/m^3 years of cumulative exposure). The investigators also noted a strong association between exposure to metalworking fluids before the ages of 23 and increased risk of prostate cancer after age 50 (RR=6.46 per 4 per 10 mg/m^3 years of cumulative exposure) suggesting that early adulthood exposures are critical to prostate cancer risk later in life.

Parkinson Disease and Trichloroethylene (TCE) Exposure

Parkinson disease (PD) is a debilitating neurodegenerative motor disorder, with its motor symptoms largely attributable to loss of dopaminergic neurons in the substantia nigra.
The causes of PD remain poorly understood, although environmental toxicants may play etiologic roles. Solvents are widespread neurotoxicants present in the workplace and ambient environment. Case reports of parkinsonism, including PD, have been associated with exposures to various solvents, most notably trichloroethylene (TCE).

Animal toxicology studies have been conducted on various organic solvents, with some, including TCE, demonstrating potential for inducing nigral system damage. Concerns about solvents possibly inducing PD have arisen from case reports of PD or clinical signs of parkinsonism during the past 20 years, mainly among exposed workers. These reports span a range of isolated cases of parkinsonism associated with various solvents, including *n*-hexane, carbon disulfide, toluene, methanol, trichloroethylene (TCE), and mixed solvents.

The largest and most extensive clinical case series investigation, conducted by Pezzoli et al. (2000) in Italy, indicated that PD patients exposed to hydrocarbon solvents (not specified by class or chemical) had earlier disease onset, more severe disease, and reduced response to treatment than did non-exposed PD patients.

The first case report of a possible link between chronic exposure to TCE and parkinsonian symptoms was in a worker who had primarily been exposed to TCE, but also had been exposed to other volatile components while working in the plastics industry. Since this initial report, the onset of PD has been reported in 3 workers chronically exposed to TCE subsequently reported an additional 3 PD cases exposed to TCE at the same small instrument plant trichloroethylene (TCE), perchloroethylene (PCE) and dichloromethane (DCM), as these have been widely used in industry. TCE and PCE given acutely to rodents, and following high exposure levels in humans are central nervous system (CNS) depressants.

Studies in mice show that repeated oral administration of TCE to rats at high doses (>0.2 g/kg/day for 6 weeks) causes depletion of dopaminergic neurons in the SNpc. While a single study in mice given high doses of TCE i.p. also resulted in loss of dopaminergic neurons in the SNpc. The scientific evidence clearly shows that high doses of TCE have the ability to damage dopaminergic neurons.

Camp Lejeune

Public Law 112-154 requires the VA to furnish hospital care and medical services to Camp Lejeune Veterans and family members with the following conditions even if there is insufficient medical evidence to conclude that such illnesses or conditions are attributable to residence at Camp Lejeune:

1. Bladder cancer
2. Breast cancer
3. Esophageal cancer
4. Female infertility
5. Hepatic steatosis
6. Kidney cancer
7. Leukemia
8. Lung cancer
9. Miscarriage
10. Multiple myeloma
11. Myelodysplastic syndromes
12. Non-Hodgkin's lymphoma
13. Neurobehavioral effects
14. Renal toxicity
15. Scleroderma

In the IOM report (page 65) the IARC concluded from sufficient evidence in animals and limited evidence in humans that PCE is probably carcinogenic in humans. Human data show a positive association between PCE and bladder cancer.

Camp Lejeune officials first realized that the drinking water supplied to some Camp Lejeune family homes may have contained volatile organic compounds ("VOCs") during routine water sampling conducted in 1980. Thereafter, in January 1982, the Navy Assessment and Control of Installation Pollutants (NACIP) program at Camp Lejeune began to identify potentially contaminated sites on the base.

Further testing later that year and in 1983 identified two VOCs: (1) trichloroethylene (TCE), a metal degreaser used for industrial purposes on the base, and (2) perchloroethylene (PCE), a dry-cleaning solvent, in two water systems serving two Camp Lejeune base housing areas. According to the National Research Council (NRC), functioning under the auspices of the National Academy of Sciences (NAS), there were multiple sources of potential pollutants.

The scientific research regarding correlations between exposure and the subsequent development of certain illnesses is still ongoing. In the meantime, veterans who were stationed at Camp Lejeune can continue to apply for service connection on a direct basis for disabilities not contemplated by the newly established presumption. In this regard, as of June 8, 2011, the Louisville, Kentucky, Regional Office (RO) (i.e., the RO at which all disability claims based on exposure to contaminated drinking water at Camp Lejeune have been consolidated) had adjudicated 125 such claims.

The weight of the evidence regarding the risk of bladder cancer associated with chlorination by-products from water disinfection continues to grow. A bladder cancer case-control study of the effects of route of exposure to trihalomethanes (ingestion through drinking water and inhalation and dermal absorption through bathing, showering and swimming in pools) found elevated risks.

Specifically, the study found that individuals living in areas with residential exposure to trihalomethanes in treated water for over 30 years have a 2-fold significant increased risk of bladder cancer. Risk was also significantly elevated among those reporting longer duration showers or baths as well as among individuals who "ever" swam in swimming pools.

New evidence regarding the risk of bladder cancer associated with solvents is primarily from a cohort study of aerospace works, which found suggestive increased risks associated with exposure to trichloroethylene (TCE) at both medium (OR=1.54) and high (OR=1.98) exposure levels, although the test for trend was not significant. In this same study, risk of bladder cancer from exposure to mineral oils was also modestly elevated, but the exposure response trend was nonmonotonic (low exposure: OR=1; medium exposure: OR=1.75; high exposure: OR=1.42). These analyses did not control for tobacco smoking, an important confounding risk factor for bladder cancer.

Based on the lifetime occupational histories of 1,129 cases of bladder cancer, a case-control study confirmed previously known or suggested links with bladder cancer, including exposure to paints and solvents, PAHs, diesel engine emissions, textiles, and aluminum production. Environmental and Occupational Causes of Cancer New Evidence, 2005–2007 Richard W. Clapp, DSc, MPH, Molly M. Jacobs, MPH, and Edward L Loechler, PhD Rev Environ Health. 2008 Jan–Mar; 23(1): 1–37.

Gulf War Syndrome

Veterans of Operation Desert Storm/Desert Shield – the 1991 Gulf War (GW) – are a unique population who returned from theater with multiple health complaints and disorders. Studies in the U.S. and elsewhere have consistently concluded that approximately 25–32% of this population suffers from a disorder characterized by symptoms that vary somewhat among individuals and include fatigue, headaches, cognitive dysfunction, musculoskeletal pain, and respiratory, gastrointestinal and dermatologic complaints.

Gulf War illness (GWI) is the term used to describe this disorder. In addition, brain cancer occurs at increased rates in subgroups of GW veterans, as do neuropsychological and brain imaging abnormalities.

Exposures in the GW theater that have been suspected of contributing to long-term health effects after the war include pesticides, depleted uranium munitions, airborne contaminants from the Kuwaiti oil well fires, chemical nerve agents, the anthrax vaccine and multiple vaccinations, widespread use of pyridostigmine bromide (PB) as a prophylactic measure against possible nerve agent exposure, chemical resistant coating (CARC) paint, and other hazards such as psychologically stressful conditions and heat.

Chemical exposures have become the focus of etiologic GWI research because nervous system symptoms are prominent and many neurotoxicants were present in theater, including organophosphates (OPs), carbamates, and other pesticides; sarin/cyclosarin nerve agents, and pyridostigmine bromide (PB) medications used as prophylaxis against chemical warfare attacks. Psychiatric etiologies have been ruled out.

Scientists concluded that exposure to pesticides and/or to PB are causally associated with GWI and the neurological dysfunction in GW veterans. Exposure to sarin and cyclosarin and to oil well fire emissions are also associated with neurologically based health effects, though their contribution to development of the disorder known as GWI is less clear.

Veterans who meet criteria for chronic multisymptom illness (CMI) must report one or more symptoms that have been ongoing for at least six months in two of three categories, which include musculoskeletal pain (symptom list: joint pain, joint stiffness, muscle pain); mood-cognition (feeling depressed, feeling moody, feeling anxious, trouble sleeping, difficulty remembering or concentrating, trouble with word finding), and fatigue. CMI can be categorized as "severe" if the veteran rates each defining symptom as severe or "mild-moderate" for milder complaints. This case definition was recommended for clinical use by a recent IOM panel.

Increased rates of migraine headaches have been reported for some time among GW deployed veterans relative to controls (Gray, Reed, Kaiser, Smith, & Gastanaga, 2002; Kang et al., 2000; Steele, 2000; Unwin et al., 1999). In GW veterans who met clinical criteria for chronic fatigue syndrome (CFS), 64% were diagnosed with migraine headaches, which is a rate similar to nonveteran subjects with CFS and significantly higher than that seen in sedentary controls (Rayhan, Ravindran, & Baraniuk, 2013).

Several studies have used functional MRI (fMRI) to assess functional anomalies and white matter integrity using diffusion tensor imaging (DTI). For example, Rayhan, Raksit, et al. (2013), Rayhan, Ravindran, et al. (2013) and Rayhan, Stevens, et al. (2013) reported that fatigue, pain and hyperalgesia were associated with diminished white matter integrity in GW veterans with CMI or CFS (Rayhan, Stevens, et al., 2013). Axial diffusivity in the right inferior fronto-occipital fasciculus specifically predicted CMI diagnosis in this study.

Toomey et al. (2009) identified differences between deployed and nondeployed veterans in a large study (N = 1061 deployed, N = 1128 nondeployed), with deployed veterans showing slower motor speed and worse attention. Also noted in this study was poorer performance on neuropsychological tests within certain domains that was associated with specific self-reported exposures. Sustained attention was poorer in veterans with self-reported exposure to contaminated food and water, verbal memory performance was worse among veterans who reported being at Khamisiyah (and presumably exposed to sarin/cyclosarin), visual memory was poorer in veterans with self-reported CARC paint exposure, and motor speed was slower among veterans who reported being near SCUD missiles (Toomey et al., 2009).

The research data to date on health in GW veterans converge to support these conclusions:

- Between one-fourth and one-third of deployed GW veterans are affected by a disorder characterized by chronic symptoms involving multiple body systems; this condition is best identified by the term GWI.
- This disorder was caused by toxicant exposures, individually or in combination, that occurred in the GW theater. At present, research most clearly and consistently links pesticide and PB exposures to GWI, while exposures to low-level nerve gas agents, contaminants from oil well fires, multiple vaccinations, and combinations of these exposures cannot be ruled out.
- In addition to GWI, deployed GW veterans suffer from a variety of neurological disorders, alone or in combination with GWI. ALS, brain cancer, stroke, migraine headaches, neuritis and neuralgia have all been reported as occurring at higher rates in this population. Rates of disorders such as MS and PD are unknown and further intensive research is needed to determine whether they are elevated in GW veterans. This should include studies focused on GW veteran subgroups classified by individual exposures or geographic locations in theater.
- Neurological disorders as well as alterations in brain structure and function have been linked to specific exposures in theater, including nerve gas agents, PB and oil well fires.

- The state of knowledge on the health of deployed GW veterans supports the conclusion that they are suffering from persistent pathology due to chemical intoxication (sometimes referred to by veterans as "toxic wounds").

CHAPTER 13 - ERECTILE DYSFUNCTION

Excerpts from Physiology of Penile Erection and Pathophysiology of Erectile Dysfunction Robert C. Dean, MD and Tom F. Lue, MD:

> "The penile erectile tissue, specifically the cavernous smooth musculature and the smooth muscles of the arteriolar and arterial walls, plays a key role in the erectile process.
>
> In the flaccid state, these smooth muscles are tonically contracted, allowing only a small amount of arterial flow for nutritional purposes. The blood partial pressure of oxygen (PO_2) is about 35mmHg range. The flaccid penis is in a moderate state of contraction, as evidenced by further shrinkage in cold weather and after phenylephrine injection.
>
> Sexual stimulation triggers release of neurotransmitters from the cavernous nerve terminals. This results in relaxation of these smooth muscles and the following events:
>
> 1. Dilatation of the arterioles and arteries by increased blood flow in both the diastolic and the systolic phases;
> 2. Trapping of the incoming blood by the expanding sinusoids;
> 3. Compression of the subtunical venular plexuses between the tunica albuginea and the peripheral sinusoids, reducing the venous outflow;

4. Stretching of the tunica to its capacity, which occludes the emissary veins between the inner circular and the outer longitudinal layers and further decreases the venous outflow to a minimum;
5. An increase in PO2 (to about 90 mmHg) and intracavernous pressure (around 100 mm Hg), which raises the penis from the dependent position to the erect state (the full-erection phase);
6. A further pressure increase (to several hundred millimeters of mercury) with contraction of the ischiocavernosus muscles (rigid-erection phase).

The innervation of the penis is both autonomic (sympathetic and parasympathetic) and somatic (sensory and motor). From the neurons in the spinal cord and peripheral ganglia, the sympathetic and parasympathetic nerves merge to form the cavernous nerves, which enter the corpora cavernosa and corpus spongiosum to affect the neurovascular events during erection and detumescence. The somatic nerves are primarily responsible for sensation and the contraction of the bulbocavernosus and ischiocavernosus muscles.

Sexual behavior and penile erection are controlled by the hypothalamus, the limbic system, and the cerebral cortex. Therefore, stimulatory or inhibitory messages can be relayed to the spinal erection centers to facilitate or inhibit erection.

It has been estimated that 10 to 19% of ED is of neurogenic origin. If one includes iatrogenic causes and mixed ED, the prevalence of neurogenic ED is probably much higher. While the presence of a neurologic disorder or neuropathy does not exclude other causes, confirming that ED is neurogenic in origin can be challenging. Because an erection is a neurovascular event, any disease or dysfunction affecting the brain, spinal cord, cavernous and pudendal nerves can induce dysfunction.

Impaired Endothelium-Dependent Vasodilatation

In patients with essential hypertension, endothelium-dependent vasodilatation, is diminished. Impairment of endothelium-dependent relaxation could be ascribed to angiotensin II thromboxane and superoxide in arteries from SHR or high blood pressure per se.

Cavernosal (Venogenic)

Failure of adequate venous occlusion has been proposed as one of the most common causes of vasculogenic impotence. Veno-occlusive dysfunction may result from the following pathophysiologic processes:

1. The presence or development of large venous channels draining the corpora cavernosa.
2. Degenerative changes (Peyronie's disease, old age, and diabetes) or traumatic injury to the

tunica albuginea (penile fracture) resulting in inadequate compression of the subtunical and emissary veins.
3. Structural alterations in the fibroelastic components of the trabeculae, cavernous smooth muscle, and endothelium may result in venous leak.
4. Insufficient trabecular smooth muscle relaxation, causing inadequate sinusoidal expansion and insufficient compression of the subtunical venules, may occur in an anxious individual with excessive adrenergic tone or in a patient with inadequate neurotransmitter release. It has been shown that alteration of an α adrenoceptor or a decrease in NO release may heighten the smooth muscle tone and impair the relaxation in response to endogenous muscle relaxant."

Erectile Dysfunction Secondary to Hypertension

A link between high blood pressure and sexual problems has been identified in men. Over time, high blood pressure damages the lining of blood vessels and causes arteries to harden and narrow (atherosclerosis), limiting blood flow. This means less blood can flow to the penis. For some men, the decreased blood flow makes it difficult to achieve and maintain erections - often referred to as erectile dysfunction. The problem is fairly common. High blood pressure can also interfere with ejaculation and reduce sexual desire. Sometimes the medications used to treat high blood pressure have similar effects.

Erectile Dysfunction Secondary to Sleep Apnea

Erectile dysfunction (ED) is quite common in men who have obstructive sleep apnea. In 2009 German researchers reported that 69% of male study participants with obstructive sleep apnea also had ED.

Men's bodies produce testosterone (a hormone that is important for sexual function) during the night. Insufficient sleep, such as that caused by sleep apnea, can reduce testosterone levels, resulting in poor erections and decreased libido.

In addition, sleep-deprived men often feel fatigued and stressed, which may worsen sexual problems. It is also possible that men with sleep apnea are not getting enough oxygen while they sleep. Oxygen is important for healthy erections, so any deficiency can cause a problem. Many men find that their erections improve with treatment of sleep apnea.

Erectile Dysfunction Secondary to PTSD

A study, *Sexual Functioning in War Veterans with Posttraumatic Stress Disorder,* by Vesna Antičević and Dolores Britvić, examined the issue of erectile dysfunction in patients with PTSD.

Posttraumatic stress disorder (PTSD) is a complex phenomenon that develops as a response to a psychological trauma and affects several levels of personality, causing changes in both mental and physical functioning. It is often associated with problems in interpersonal relationships and difficulties with attachment, intimacy, and sexuality. Problems in the realm of sexuality arise from the individual's inability to establish an adequate emotional-physical relationship with the partner, as well as from the disturbances in mental and physical health.

Several studies found that the prevalence of sexual dysfunctions among patients with PTSD was higher than in general population. Dysfunctions can occur in almost all domains of sexuality – activity, desire, arousal, orgasm, and satisfaction with sexual life. The most frequent difficulties are erectile dysfunction and premature ejaculation. Antidepressant therapy is an additional factor that can aggravate difficulties in sexual functioning.

Vesna Antičević et al. found lower sexual desire, lower frequency of sexual activities, and a more frequent erectile dysfunction and painful intercourse in respondents with PTSD than in controls. Reduced sexual desire was more prominent in veterans with PTSD who were taking antidepressant therapy (except on the variable of masturbation) than in those who were not taking it, whereas premature ejaculation was more frequent in veterans who were not taking antidepressants than in those who were. This study's findings can also be compared with the findings of studies conducted in the US, Korea, and Israel.

Diabetes is an Established Risk Factor for Sexual Dysfunction

Diabetes is an established risk factor for sexual dysfunction in men; a threefold increased risk of erectile dysfunction was documented in diabetic men, as compared with nondiabetic men.

Hyperglycemia, which is a main determinant of vascular and microvascular diabetic complications, may participate in the pathogenetic mechanisms of sexual dysfunction in diabetes. Moreover, diabetic people may present several clinical conditions, including hypertension, overweight and obesity, metabolic syndrome, cigarette smoking, and atherogenic dyslipidemia, which are themselves risk factors for sexual dysfunction, both in men and in women

Epidemiological studies suggest that both type 1 and type 2 diabetes are associated with an increased risk of ED, which is reported to occur in ≥50% of men with diabetes worldwide. In the Massachusetts, Male Aging Study, diabetic men showed a threefold probability of having ED when compared to men without diabetes; moreover, the age-adjusted risk of ED doubled in diabetic men when compared to those without diabetes.

The proposed mechanisms of ED in diabetic patients are represented by vasculopathy, neuropathy, visceral adiposity, insulin resistance, and hypogonadism.

Diabetic vasculopathy concerns macroangiopathy, microangiopathy, and endothelial dysfunction. Macrovascular disease in diabetes corresponds to the atherosclerotic damage in the blood vessels, which limits blood flow to the penis. As mentioned, several cardiovascular risk factors associated with diabetes contribute to the genesis of penile arterial insufficiency: all of them converge on endothelial dysfunction, which represents the common denominator leading to vascular ED.
Microvascular disease determines ischemic damage in the distal circulation and autonomic and peripheral neuropathy. Both somatic and autonomic neuropathies may contribute to diabetes-induced ED due to the impairment of sensory impulses from the penis to the reflexogenic erectile center, and reduced or absent parasympathetic activity necessary for relaxation of the smooth muscle of the corpus cavernosum.

Insulin resistance and visceral adiposity, which are both distinctive clinical traits of type 2 diabetes, are associated with a proinflammatory state that results in the decreased availability and activity of NO, leading to ED in overweight and obese diabetic men.

CHAPTER 14 - CLAIMS FOR DISABILITY DUE TO VA NEGLIGENT CARE PURSUANT TO 38 U.S.C.S. 1151

Section 1151 authorizes the VA to treat disabilities or death resulting from VA hospital care as service-connected. Section 1151 requires that injury or death be proximately caused by carelessness, negligence, lack of proper skill, error in judgment, or similar instance of fault or by an event not reasonably foreseeable. The statute disallows compensation in all cases where disability or death resulted from the veteran's willful misconduct.

The VA's regulatory requirements are in line with civil medical malpractice standards, which typically consider how a reasonable health care provider would have acted under the circumstances and require a showing of proximate cause. The primary difference between a civil medical malpractice case and a Section 1151 claim is the lower standard of proof applicable to VA claims. The standard of proof in most civil cases, including medical malpractice cases, is the preponderance of the evidence standard. For VA claims, the standard of proof is lower –- the benefit-of-the-doubt. Thus, in order to prevail on any issue material to a 1151 claim a claimant need only show that the positive and negative evidence is in approximate balance.

Section 1151 explicitly requires that VA care cause the disability or death and that the VA fault or accident be the proximate cause of the disability or death. VA regulations define proximate cause as the action or event that directly caused the disability or death, as distinguished from a remote contributing cause. VA regulations provide that actual causation must be shown. The fact that a veteran received VA care and now has additional disability or has died is not sufficient to establish causation.

VA regulations provide multiple means to establish that VA medical care, treatment, or examination proximately caused disability or death. The claimant can show:

- VA failed to exercise the degree of care that would be expected of a reasonable health care provider; or
- VA furnished the care without the veterans, or his or her surrogates, informed consent; or
- The event was not reasonably foreseeable based on what a reasonable health care provider would have foreseen.

Informed consent is defined as freely given consent that follows a careful explanation by the practitioner to the patient or the patient's surrogate of the proposed diagnostic or therapeutic procedure or course of treatment. The practitioner must explain the treatment in understandable language and discuss the expected benefits, reasonably foreseeable associated risks, complications or side effects, reasonable and available alternatives, and anticipated results if no action is taken.

There must be an opportunity to ask questions, to indicate comprehension of the information, and to grant permission freely without coercion. The VA Manual indicates that express consent is consent that has been clearly stated either orally or in writing.

Under 38 C.F.R. 17.32(b), consent may be implied rather than expressed. Consent is implied when immediate medical care is necessary to preserve life or prevent serious impairment of the health of the patient or others, and the patient is unable to consent, and the practitioner determines that the there is no surrogate or that waiting for consent from a surrogate would increase the hazard to the life or health of the patient or others.

The VA determines whether an event was not reasonably foreseeable based on what a reasonable health care provider would have foreseen. The event does not need to be completely unforeseeable or unimaginable, but it must be one that a reasonable health care provider would not consider an ordinary treatment risk. Relevant to this issue is whether the event was the type that a reasonable health care provider would have disclosed in connection with informed consent procedures. Therefore, when informed consent documents fail to mention the event that resulted in the disability or death, they provide support that the event was not reasonably foreseeable.

The degree of deviation from the standard of care is not as high as is required in a typical medical malpractice case.

As with any claim, when there is an approximate balance of positive and negative evidence regarding any matter material to the claim, the claimant shall be given the benefit of the doubt 38 USCA §5107 (West 2002). To establish causation, evidence must show that the hospital care, medical or surgical treatment, or examination resulted in the veteran's additional disability or death. The degree of deviation from the standard of care is not as high as is required in a typical medical malpractice case. The veteran merely needs to show that it is as likely as not that the care provided was less than the required standard of care.

In *Jackson v. Nicholson,* 433. F.3d. 822 (Fed. Cir. 2005). The Federal Circuit Court determined that the injury need not be a result of the fault or action of VA personnel; the fact that an injury occurred as a circumstance of being in the hospital was enough to establish the causation requirement for compensation purposes (Id. at 825-26). Most recently, the Board relying on the Federal Circuit Court in the case of *Viegas v. Shinseki,* 2012-7075, 2013 WL 363004 (Fed. Cir. January 31, 2013), held that a veteran who died in the hospital from aspergillus infection was entitled to disability benefits pursuant to § 1151 even though the claimant was unable to show the precise mechanism through which he acquired the infection.

In *Viegas* the Court held:

> "A similar analysis applies here. Although the government asserts that a veteran's disability must be 'directly' caused by the provision of hospital care or medical treatment, section 1151 contains not "so much as a word about" direct causation. There is simply nothing in the plain language of the statute, which requires that an injury be 'directly' caused by the medical care provided by VA personnel. Instead, the statute requires only a "causal connection," Gardner, 513 U.S. at 119, between the injuries sustained by the veteran and the hospital care or medical treatment provided by the VA."

CHAPTER 15 – PROPOSED REDUCTION IN VA BENEFITS

Once a veteran is granted disability benefits, the VA will routinely re-examine the veteran to determine whether there has been any improvement in his/her condition since the award of benefits. If the VA finds that there has been an improvement, they will provide a veteran with a proposed plan for reduction of benefits. The veteran is advised that he/she needs to provide new medical records to negate a reduction in benefits.

The proposed reduction is not considered an actual denial of benefits, and therefore, veterans are not allowed to have an attorney assist them at this stage. It is, however, crucial that the veteran object to the reduction in benefits and provide a rebuttal to the VA's allegation and examination by an experienced physician, ideally in the form of an Independent Medical Opinion (IMO).

Unlike other administrative actions, a reduction in a veteran's disability evaluation is not permitted merely because a later adjudicator has a different opinion on how the evidence or the rating schedule should be interpreted. A reduction in a veteran's disability rating is permitted only where certain circumstances exist, and where particular legal guidelines have been satisfied. *Dofflemyer*, 2 Vet. App. at 280, *Cushman v. Shinseki*, 576 F.3d 1290 (Fed. Cir. 2009). Before any existing disability evaluation can be lawfully reduced, the VA is obligated to satisfy a variety of legal requirements.

Moreover, the VA bears the burden of proof in establishing, by a preponderance of the evidence, that a reduction is warranted under the relevant regulations. See *Hayes*, 9 Vet. App. at 73; *Kitchens v. Brown*, 7 Vet. App. 320, 325 (1995); *Brown v. Brown*, 5 Vet. App. 413, 421 (1993). Veterans who have been assigned 100% schedular evaluations or 100% evaluations based on individual unemployability, or veterans who have had ratings that have been in effect for five years or more, receive special protection.

The Requirement of Sustained Improvement to Reduce a Rating Level That Has Been in Effect for Five or More Years

Any rating evaluation that has stabilized, for five years or more may not be reduced unless all the evidence of record shows sustained improvement in the disability. 38 C.F.R. 3.344(c) (2011). Because 38 C.F.R. 3.344(a) requires that all the evidence of record support the conclusion that sustained improvement in the disability has occurred, the VA cannot view the single examination upon which the reduction is proposed in isolation from the rest of the record. *Schafrath*, 1 Vet. App. at 594. *See also* VA Fast Letter 10-14 Revised (July 29, 2010). In other words, the entire medical history of the disability must always be considered in conjunction with any rating examination upon which a reduction is proposed. *See also Brown*, 5 Vet. App. at 421. In *Schafrath v. Derwinski*, the court explained the purpose of this rule as follows:

"These requirements for evaluation of the complete medical history of the claimant's condition operate to protect claimants against adverse decisions based on a single, incomplete or inaccurate report and to enable VA to make a more precise evaluation of the level of the disability and of any changes in the condition. These considerations are especially strong in a ratings reduction case." *Schafrath*, 1 Vet. App. at 594

The *Schafrath* Court emphasized:

"It is precisely because a disability is stabilized that the VA must take care when proposing to reduce the rating evaluation assigned to it. Because [s]uch disabilities are considered stabilized...the regulation thus requires a high degree of accuracy in decisions reducing those ratings." *Schafrath*, 1 Vet. App. at 594

To meet its duty under 38 C.F.R. 3.344(a), the VA must review the entire record of examinations and the medical-industrial history in order to ascertain whether the recent examination [upon which the VA is relying to reduce the rating] is full and complete. *Brown*, 5 Vet. App. at 419 (citing 38 C.F.R. 3.344(a)). Any examination that is less full and complete than that examination on which payments were authorized or continued may not be used as a basis of reduction. 38

C.F.R. 3.344(a). If the disability is subject to temporary and episodic improvement, it will not be reduced on any one examination, except in those circumstances in which all the evidence of record clearly warrants the conclusion that sustained improvement has been demonstrated. 38 C.F.R. 3.344(a). Even though material improvement in the physical or mental condition is clearly demonstrated, the VA will [consider] whether the evidence makes it reasonably certain that the improvement will be maintained under the ordinary conditions of life. 38 C.F.R. 3.344(a).

Rules Regulating the Reduction of Total (100%) Disability Evaluations

When the VA considers reducing a total (100%) rating, the issue to be decided is not whether the veteran's current symptomatology is equal to the symptomatology needed for the 100% evaluation. *See Dofflemyer*, 2 Vet. App. at 279-80. Rather the VA must decide whether there has been material improvement in the physical or mental condition evaluated as 100% disabling. 38 C.F.R. 3.343(a) (2011). Without an examination that confirms such improvement, the VA is prohibited from reducing the veteran's rating. 38 C.F.R. 3.343(a)

In *Karnas v. Derwinski*, 1 Vet. App. 308 (1991), the CAVC ruled that if there has been no improvement at all since the date of the last examination continuing the 100% rating, a reduction is prohibited. When deciding whether there has been improvement in the veteran's condition, the CAVC has held that the VA may look at both medical and nonmedical evidence to determine whether a veteran's condition has materially improved. *Faust v. West*, 13 Vet. App. 342, 349-50 (2000).

If the VA determines that a reduction in a total schedular rating (100%) is warranted, but the record reflects that the veteran is unable to engage in substantially gainful employment by virtue of his or her service-connected disability, the veteran must be awarded a total (100%) rating based on the individual unemployability (TDIU) provisions of 38 C.F.R. 4.16.604. Moreover, once a veteran is in receipt of benefits at the total rating level based on TDIU, the VA may not reduce the benefits unless clear and convincing evidence establishes that the veteran is capable of actual employment. 38 C.F.R. 3.343(c) (2011). *See Faust*, 13 Vet. App. at 356.

In a similar case recently decided by the Board, (Citation Nr: 1203550, Decision Date: 01/31/12, DOCKET NO. 05-15 764, Archive Date: 02/07/12), the Board recognized that since there was no evidence for a recurrence of the cancer, 100% disability was not appropriate based on the specific rating code. Yet the Board held that remand was necessary to ascertain whether the veteran's status of total unemployability must also be changed such that the effect of the cancer and the anticancer treatment had dissipated allowing the veteran to work. The Board held:

> "A claim for entitlement to a total rating based on individual unemployability due to service-connected disability (TDIU) is part of an increased rating issue when such

claim is raised by the record and the Board has jurisdiction over the issue of TDIU because it is part of the claim for increased compensation. *Rice v. Shinseki*, 22 Vet. App. 447 (2009). At his February 2010 VA examination, the Veteran indicated that he could only work 2 hours a day due to fatigue, and at his October 2010 VA examination the Veteran essentially asserted that he had missed 32 weeks of work the prior 12 months due to fatigue and depression (the Veteran is service-connected for PTSD). Entitlement to a TDIU has not been adjudicated by the AOJ. As such, it must be adjudicated by the AOJ prior to appellate consideration.

Accordingly, the case is REMANDED for the following action:

1. Issue VCAA notice relative to the issue of entitlement to a TDIU.

2. Undertake any other necessary development and then adjudicate the issue of entitlement to a TDIU rating. If the benefit sought is not granted, the Veteran and his representative should be furnished with a Supplemental Statement of the Case, and afforded a reasonable opportunity to respond before the record is returned to the Board for further review.

The Veteran has the right to submit additional evidence and argument on the matter the Board has remanded. *Kutscherousky v. West*, 12 Vet. App. 369 (1999)."

Appendix A – David Anaise, MD, JD Curriculum Vitae

David Anaise, MD, JD

CURRICULUM VITAE

EDUCATION AND TRAINING:

- Hebrew University, Hadassah Medical School, Jerusalem, Israel, M.D. 1975
- Resident in General Surgery, SUNY at Stony Brook, New York 1976-1981
- Transplantation Fellowship SUNY at Stony Brook, New York 1981-1982
- American Board of Surgery Certification #037547, December 3, 1982
- American Board of Surgery Recertified October 1998
- Licensed in Maryland
- University of Arizona College of Law JD May 1999

HOSPITAL AND ACADEMIC APPOINTMENTS:

- Assistant Clinical Professor Department of Surgery George Washington University Washington DC 1992- present
- Attending Surgeon General Surgery and Transplantation Washington Hospital Center Washington DC 1992- 1996
- Senior staff surgeon Henry Ford Hospital Detroit MI 1991-1992
- Medical director transplantation services Sierra Medical Center El Paso Texas 1989-1991
- Clinical Associate Professor in Surgery, Attending Surgeon in Transplantation and General Surgery Department of Surgery, SUNY at Stony Brook, New York 11794 1982-1989

MEMBERSHIP IN PROFESSIONAL SOCIETIES:

- The Transplantation Society

- American Society of Transplant Surgeons
- European Society for Organ Transplantation
- Fellow, American College of Surgeons

HONORS:

- Assistant Editor, Transplantation Proceedings
- President, New York Transplantation Society, 1988-1989
- Representative of the State of New York to the Organ Procurement and
- Distribution Committee of the United Network for Organ Sharing (UNOS)
- Board of Directors New York Regional Transplant Program (NYRTP)

MILITARY SERVICE:

Captain, Israeli Medical Corps. 1971-1974

PERSONAL:

Born 2/12/46 Jerusalem Israel

PATENTS:

- U.S. Patent #4,723,939. Apparatus & Methods for Multiple organ procurement
- U.S. Patent #309,288 Method for hypothermic organ protection during organ procurement from non - heart beating cadaver donors
- U.S Patent # 576,058 Hemostatic Organ Preservation System

BOOK CHAPTERS:

David Anaise: Pharmacologic Agents in Organ Preservation
In: "Procurement and Preservation of Vascularized Organs"
G. M. Collins Editor Klwer Academic Publisher 1996

David Anaise: Salvage of Organs from Non Heart-Beating Cadaver Donors

In: "Procuring Organs for Transplant"
R. M Arnold MD editor John Hopkins University Press 1996

David Anaise, Mark Yland: Perfusion and Storage Techniques
In: "Basic Concepts of Organ Procurement"
L Toledo Peryera MD Editor RG Landes Co 1996

David Anaise The technology of transplantation
In: "Bioethics and Law"
Michael H Shapiro and Roy G. Spece Jr. editors West publication 2003

PUBLICATIONS:

106 articles published in peer reviewed journals

BIBLIOGRAPHY:

1. Ben-Hur, N., Golan, Y. and Anaise, D. Reimplantation of four amputated fingers using microsurgical technique. Harefua, D:81, 1976.
2. Eldad, A., Stark, M. and Anaise, D. Amniotic membranes as a biological dressing in the treatment of burns. S. African Med. J., 51:272, 1977.
3. Anaise, D., Steinitz, R. and Ben-Hur, N. Solar radiation as a possible etiologic factor in malignant melanoma. Cancer, 42:299, 1978.
4. Anaise, D. and Hines, G. L. Limb salvage by use of an extra-anatomical bypass. Med. J. Nassau Hosp., 3:5, 1981.
5. Golan, J., Anaise, D. and Eylath, U. Treatment of cutaneous malignant melanoma in Israel, 1960-1970. Ann. Plastic Surg., 8:397, 1982.
6. Anaise, D., Atkins, H. and Oster, A. Non -invasive radionucleide scintiphotography technique for the assessment of preserved renal allograft
viability. J. Nucl. Med., 24:15, 1983.
7. Anaise, D., Atkins, H., Asari, H., Oster, Z., Waltzer, W.C., Bachvaroff, R.J. and Rapaport, F.T. Pretransplant assessment of preserved renal allograft viability by radionuclide scintiphotography. Fed. Proc., 42:1088, 1983.
8. Asari, H., Anaise, D., Bachvaroff, R.J. and Rapaport, F.T. Protective effects of a calmodulin inhibitor in canine kidney preservation. Fed. Proc., 42:1088, 1983.
9. Waltzer, W.C., Bachvaroff, R.J., Anaise, D., Raisbeck, A.P., Asari, H. and Rapaport, F.T. Parameters of immunological reactivity in patients with end –stage renal disease (ESRD) awaiting transplantation. Fed. Proc., 42:941, 1983.
10. Waltzer, W.C., Anaise, D., Asari, H . and Rapaport, F.T. Management of urological transplant complications by utilization of the host ureter. Transpl.

Proc., 15:2152, 1983.
11. Asari, H., Anaise, D., Bachvaroff, R.J. and Rapaport, F.T. Usefulness of trifluoperazine in canine kidney preservation. Transp. Proc., 16:184, 1984.
12. Anaise, D., Brandt, D. and Smith, N. Pitfalls in the diagnosis and treatment of gastric diverticulum. Gastrointestinal Endoscopy, 30:28, 1984.
13. Anaise, D., Atkins, H., Asari, H. Oster, Z., Waltzer, W.C., Bachvaroff, R.J. and Rapaport, F.T. A non-invasive approach to the assessment of organ viability after kidney preservation in dogs. Transpl. Proc., 16:164, 1984.
14. Asari, H., Anaise, D., Bachvaroff, R.J., Sato, T. and Rapaport, F.T. Preservation techniques for organ transplantation. I. Protective effects of calmodulin inhibitors in cold-preserved kidneys. Transpl., 37:113, 1984.
15. Anaise, D., Asari, H., Sato, K., Waltzer, W.C., Bachvaroff, R.J., Oster, Z., Atkins, H. and Rapaport, F.T. The beneficial effect of trifluoperazine (TFP) on the microcirculation and subsequent function of the cold preserved kidney. Transpl. Proc., 16:1333, 1984.
16. Waltzer, W.C., Bachvaroff, R.J., Anaise, D. and Rapaport, F.T. Natural killer activity after renal transplantation. Transpl. Proc., 16:1527, 1984.
17. Waltzer, W.C., Bachvaroff, R.J., Anaise, D. and Rapaport, F.T. Lymphocyte subpopulations in renal transplantation. Transpl. Proc., 16:1554, 1984.
18. Waltzer, W.C., Bachvaroff, R.J., Shen, L., Anaise, D. and Rapaport, F.T. Human Natural Killer (NK) cell activity in kidney allograft recipients. Fed. Proc., 43:663, 1984.
19. Waltzer, W.C., Frischer, Z., Anaise, D., Sato, K. and Rapaport, F.T. Restoration of urinary tract continuity after necrosis of the pelvis and ureter in a transplanted kidney - the boari flap. Transpl. Proc., 16:1367, 1984.
20. Anaise, D., Waltzer, W.C., Sato, K., Frischer, Z. and Rapaport, F.T. Usefulness of the Dennis tube for in situ cold perfusion of cadaver donor kidneys. Transpl. Proc., 16:1661, 1984.
21. Anaise, D., Cottrell, T., Ellis, P., Waltzer, W. and Rapaport, F.T. Biliary stenosis secondary to pancreatitis - an unusual cause of obstructive jaundice in a renal transplant recipient. Transpl. Proc., 16:1669, 1984.
22. Waltzer, W.C., Bachvaroff, R.J., Anaise, D. and Rapaport, F.T. Lymphocyte subpopulations in patients with end-stage renal disease (ESRD). Abstracts of the IXth Inti. Congress of Nephrology, Los Angeles, California, June 11-16, 1984, p.305A.
23. Shen, L., Waltzer, W.C., Anaise, D., Bachvaroff, R.J. and Rapaport, F.T. The value of monitoring T-lymphocyte subpopulations after kidney transplantation. Fed. Proc., 43:609, 1984.
24. Waltzer, W.C., Anaise, D., Frischer, Z. and Rapaport, F.T. Renal transplantation and Boeck 's sarcoidosis. Transpl. Proc., 16:1359, 1984.
25. Waltzer, W.C., Anaise, D., Arbeit, L., Weinstein, S. and Rapaport, F.T. Usefulness of Captopril in the management of hypertension after renal

transplantation. Transpl. Proc., 16:1372, 1984.
26. Anaise, D., Sato, K., Atkins, H., Oster, Z., Asari, H., Waltzer, W.C., Pollack, W., Bachvaroff, R.J. and Rapaport, F.T. Scintigraphic evaluation of the viability of cold preserved kidneys prior to transplantation. J. Nuclear Med., 25:1304, 1984.
27. Anaise, D., Bachvaroff, R.J., Sato, K., Waltzer, W.C., Asari, H., Pollack, W., Oster, Z., Atkins, H. and Rapaport, F.T. Enhanced resistance to the effects of hypothermic ischemia in the preserved canine kidney. Transpl., 38:570, 1984.
28. Anaise, D., Sato, K., Waltzer, W.C., Bachvaroff, R.J., Oster, Z., Atkins, H., Pollack, W. and Rapaport, F.T. A membrane stabilization approach to long-term renal preservation. Transpl. Proc., 17:1457, 1984.
29. Waltzer, W.C., Arnold, A., Anaise, D. and Rapaport, F.T. Human natural killer (NK) cell activity following renal transplantation. Abstracts of the 80th Annual Convention of the American Urological Association, Atlanta, Georgia, May 12-16, 1985. p. 232A.
30. Waltzer, W.C., Arnold, A., Anaise, D. and Rapaport, F.T. Monitoring of T-cell subpopulations following renal transplantation. Abstracts of the 80th Annual Convention of the American Urological Association, Atlanta, Georgia, May 12-lb, 1985. p. 232A.
31. Waltzer, W.C., Frischer, Z., Anaise, D., Sato, K. and Rapaport, F.T. Management of bladder neck contracture at the time of renal transplantation. Transpl. Proc., 17:2009, 1985.
32. Waltzer, W.C., Bachvaroff, R.J., Arnold, A., Anaise, D. and Rapaport, F.T. Immunological consequence of renal transplantation and immunosuppression. I. Alterations in human natural killer cell activity. J. Clin. Immunol., 5:78, 1985.
33. Waltzer, W.C., Anaise, D., Gonda, A.C., Sato, K. and Rapaport, F.T. Use of self-retained coiled silicone stent for management of recurrent transplant ureteral stricture. Transpl. Proc., 17:2016, 1985.
34. Waltzer, W.C., Anaise, D., Sato, K., Atkins, H., Oster, Z., Cavallaro, D., Miller, F. and Rapaport, F.T. Acute lymphedema in a renal allograft - an unusual cause of early post-operative transplant dysfunction. Transpl. Proc., 17:1755, 1985.
35. Waltzer, W.C., Anaise, D., Arbeit, L. A., Miller, F., Weinstein, S. W., and Rapaport, F.T. Allograft rejection and the nephrotic syndrome. Transpl. Proc., 17:1763, 1985.
36. Atkins, H. L., Oster, Z. H., Anaise, D., Weis, S., Waltzer, W.C., Gonda, A., Cooch, E., and Rapaport, F.T. Cortical perfusion index - a predictor of acute rejection in transplanted kidneys. J. Nucl. Med., 26:132, 1985.
37. Waltzer, W.C., Arnold, A.N., Anaise, D., Lehr, H.A., and Rapaport, F.T. A comparison of the effects of cyclosporine and azathioprine on human natural killer (NK) activity in renal allograft recipients. Transpl. Proc., 17:2719, 1985.
38. Lehr, H., Jao, S., Waltzer, W.C., Anaise, D. and Rapaport, F. T.

Cytomegalovirus-induced diabetes mellitus in a renal allograft recipient. Transpl. Proc., 17:2152, 1985.
39. Waltzer, W.C., Gonda, A., Lehr, H., Anaise, D., Frischer, Z. and Rapaport, F.T. Management of transplant ureteropelvic junction obstruction by dismembered pyeloplasty. Transpl. Proc., 17:2149, 1985.
40. Arnold, A. N., Waltzer, W.C., Anaise, D., Weinstein, S. W., and Rapaport, F.T. Effect of renal allograft dysfunction upon cyclosporine trough levels in host blood. Transpl., 40:605, 1985.
41. Lehr, H.A., Bairn, R.S., Waltzer, W.C., Anaise, D. and Rapaport, F.T. Comparative efficacy of ultrasound and core needle biopsy techniques for the differential diagnosis of acute renal allograft rejection crises. Transpl. Proc., 18:1057, 1986.
42. Anaise, D., Atkins, H., Oster, Z., Weis, S., Gonda, A., Waltzer, W.C., and Rapaport, F.T. Use of renal cortex perfusion indices for the diagnosis of acute allograft rejection crises. Transpl. Proc. 18:1048, 1986.
43. Lehr, H.A., Waltzer, W.C., Anaise, D., and Rapaport, F.T. Management of a post-biopsy arterial pseudoaneurysm in a transplanted kidney: utilization of epsilon aminocaproic acid and controlled hypotension. Transpl. Proc., 18:976, 1986.
44. Kimmelstiel, F., Anaise, D., Waltzer, W.C., Arnold, A.N., and Rapaport, F.T. Radionuclide scans and needle biopsies in the diagnosis and treatment of renal allograft pyelonephritis and rejection developing during post-operative acute tubular necrosis. Transpl. Proc., 18:963, 1986.
45. Anaise, D., Waltzer, W.C., and Rapaport, F.T. Metabolic requirements for successful extended hypothermic kidney preservation. J. Urol., 136:345, 1986.
46. Anaise, D., Oster, Z.H., Atkins, H.L., Arnold, A. N., Weis, S., Waltzer, W.C., and Rapaport, F.T. Cortex perfusion index - a sensitive detector of acute rejection crisis in transplanted kidneys. J. Nuclear Med., 27:1697, 1986.
47. Waltzer, W.C., Arnold, A.N., Anaise, D., and Rapaport, F.T. A comparison of immune profiles in Cyclosporine- and Azathioprine-treated renal allograft recipients. Transpl. Proc. 18:1332, 1986.
48. Prives, J., Anaise, D., Lane, B. and Rapaport, F.T. Adverse effects of angiotensin and calmodulin on the vascular smooth muscle of the cold preserved kidney. The Physiologist, 29:116, 1986.
49. Anaise, D., Ramsammy, L, Lane, B. and Rapaport, F.T. Do calcium inhibitors prevent free radicals' release during prolonged hypothermic renal ischemia? The Physiologist, 29:161, 1986.
50. Greif, F., Anaise, D., Arbeit, L., Frei, L., and Soroff, H.S. Inhibition of the calcium cascade in renal ischemia. The Physiologist, 29:116, 1986.
51. Waltzer, W.C., Arnold, A., Anaise, D. and Rapaport, F.T. Contrasting results of immunological monitoring in cyclosporine and azathioprine treated renal allograft recipients. Transpl. Proc., 18:970, 1986.
52. Sato, K., Asari, H., Masaki, Y., Nakayama, Y., Yokota, K. Uchida, H., Aso, K., Anaise, D., Waltzer, W.C. and Rapaport, F.T. Successful 72, 96

and 120 hour preservation of the canine kidney by using simple surface cooling with Trifluoperazine (TFP), high dose Urokinase, Verapamil and modified Collins' solution. Low Temp. Med., 12:14, 1986.
53. Greif, F., Anaise, D., Frei, L., Arbeit, L., and Soroff, H. Role of calcium antagonists in averting acute tubular necrosis after prolonged renal ischemia. Surgical Forum, 37:64, 1986.
54. Waltzer, W.C., Miller, F., Arnold, A., Anaise, D. and Rapaport, F.T. Immunologic and clinical evaluation of renal allograft dysfunction by percutaneous core biopsy. Abstracts of the 82nd Annual Convention of the American Urological Association, Anaheim, California, May 17-21, 1987. p.245A.
55. Waltzer, W.C., Arnold, A., Anaise, D. and Rapaport, F.T. Impact of cytomegalovirus infection and HLA matching on rejection following renal transplantation. Abstracts of the 82nd Annual Convention of the American Urological Association, Anaheim, California, May 17-21, 1987. p. 324A.
56. Anaise, D., Lane, B., Waltzer, W.C., Rapaport, F.T. The protective effect of calcium inhibitors and of captopril on the renal microcirculation during reperfusion. Transpl., 43:128, 1987.
57. Anaise, D., Waltzer, W.C., Arnold, A., and Rapaport, F.T. Adverse effects of Cyclosporin A on the microcirculation of the cold preserved kidney. N.Y.S J. Med., 87:141, 1987.
58. Waltzer, W.C., Miller, F., Arnold, A., Anaise, D., and Rapaport, F.T. Immunohistologic analysis of human renal allograft dysfunction. Transpl., 43:100, 1987.
59. Anaise, D., Lehr, H., Atkins, H., Oster, Z., Arnold, A., Waltzer, W.C., and Rapaport, F.T. Preservation of the cortical renal microcirculation - a prerequisite for immediate renal allograft function. Transpl. Proc., 19:2039, 1987.
60. Pullis, C.K., Waltzer, W.C., Arnold, A. N., Anaise, D.A., and Rapaport, F.T. Differential effects of cyclosporine and azathioprine on host cell populations in renal allograft recipients. Transpl. Proc., 19:1596, 1987.
61. Waltzer, W.C., Miller, F., Arnold, A.N., Anaise, D. and Rapaport, F.T. Identification of mononuclear cell populations infiltrating human renal allografts. Transpl. Proc., 19:1629, 1987.
62. Anaise, D., Ramsammy, L., Lane, B., Waltzer, W.C. and Rapaport, F.T. The Pathophysiology of the no-reflow phenomenon in cold stored kidneys. Transpl. Proc., 19:1348, 1987.
63. Sato, K., Asari, H., Masaki, Y., Uchida, H., Aso, K., Yoda, Y., Ishii, K., Anaise, D., Waltzer, W.C. and Rapaport, F.T. Usefulness of radionuclide scintiphotography to evaluate preserved kidney viability. Transpl. Proc., 19: 2043, 1987.
64. Asari, H., Sato, K., Sonoda, K., Uchida, H., Ishihara, A., Anaise, D. and

Rapaport, F.T. Protective effects of calmodulin inhibitor in canine kidney preservation. Transpl. Proc., 19:1363, 1987.
65. Arnold, A., Anaise, D., Miller, F., Waltzer, W.C. and Rapaport, F.T. Prevention of chronic rejection by cyclosporine and prednisone. Transpl. Proc., 19:2122, 1987.
66. Waltzer, W.C., Miller, F., Arnold, A.N., Jao, S., Anaise, D. and Rapaport, F.T. Value of percutaneous core needle biopsy in the differential diagnosis of renal transplant dysfunction. J. Urology, 137:1117, 1987.
67. Anaise, D., Yland, M.J., Waltzer, W.C., Frischer, Z., and Rapaport, F.T. A new perfusion tube for multiple organ procurement. Transpl. Proc., 19:4129, 1987.
68. Anaise, D., Yland, M.J., Atkins, H.L., Oster, Z.H., Waltzer, W.C., and Rapaport, F.T. Additive effects of cyclosporine and cold preservation upon the integrity of the renal cortical microcirculation. Transpl. Proc., 19:3606, 1987.
69. Atkins, H.L., Anaise, D., Oster, Z.H., Yland, M.J., Waltzer, W.C., and Rapaport, F.T. The evaluation of cold-storage and immunosuppression of renal allografts by using the cortical perfusion index. J. Nuclear Medicine, 28:731, 1987.
70. Kubota, K., Atkins, H. L., Anaise, D., Oster, Z.H., and Pollack, W. Quantitative evaluation of renal excretion on the dynamic DTPA renal scan. J. Nuclear Medicine, 28:733, 1987.
71. Waltzer, W.C., Arnold, A.N., Anaise, D., Hurley, S., Raisbeck, A., Egelandsdsdal, B., Pullis, C. and Rapaport, F.T. Impact of cytomegalovirus
infection and HLA-matching on outcome of renal transplantation. Transpl. Proc., 19:4077, 1987.
72. Oster, Z.H., Bazin, J.P., Raynaud, C., Anaise, D., Di Paola, M., Di Paola, R., Rapaport, F.T., and Atkins, H.L. Renal transplant (RT) evaluation with Tc-99m DTPA (DTPA) - The role of factorial analysis. J. Nuclear Medicine, 28:680, 1987.
73. Waltzer, W.C., Shabtai, M., Anaise, D. and Rapaport, F.T. Usefulness and limitations of Doppler ultrasonography in the evaluation of post-operative renal allograft dysfunction. Abstracts of the 83rd Annual Convention of the American Urological Association, Boston, Massachusetts, June 3-7, 1988. p. 232A.
74. Waltzer, W.C., Shabtai, M., Frischer, Z., Anaise, D. and Rapaport, F.T. Early aggressive management for the prevention of renal allograft loss and patient mortality following major urological complications. Abstracts of the 83rd Annual Convention of the American Urological Association, Boston, Massachusetts, June 3-7, 1988. p. 418A.
75. Kimmelstiel, F., Anaise, D., Waltzer, W.C., and Rapaport, F.T. Continuous post-operative peritoneal lavage for the management of intra-abdominal sepsis in renal allograft recipients. Transpl. Proc., 20:101, 1988.

76. Shabtai, M., Luft, B., Waltzer, W.C., Anaise, D., and Rapaport, F.T. Massive cytomegalovirus pneumonia and myocarditis in a renal transplant recipient - successful treatment with DHPG. Transpl. Proc., 20:562, 1988.
77. Waltzer, W.C., Miller, F., Arnold, A.N., Anaise, D., and Rapaport, F.T. Immunological analysis of cellular infiltrates during human renal allograft dysfunction. Transpl. Proc., 20:111, 1988.
78. Anaise, D., Yland, M.J., Waltzer, W.C., Frischer, Z., Hurley, S., Eychmueller, S., and Rapaport, F.T. Flush pressure requirements for optimal cadaveric donor kidney preservation. Transpl. Proc., 20:891, 1988.
79. Yland, M.J., Anaise, D., Kimmelstiel, F., Eychmueller, S., Romano, E., Waltzer, W.C., Frischer, Z., and Rapaport, F.T. The usefulness of initial brief pulsatile perfusion (BPP) in extending the applicability of cold storage for renal transplantation - a preliminary report. Transpl. Proc., 20:875, 1988.
80. Marks, L.A., Anaise, D., and Yland, M.J. Renal admittance plethysmosgraphy. Proceedings of the 14th Annual Northeast Bioengineering Conference, March 10-11, 1988.
81. Shabtai, M., Waltzer, W.C., Miller, F., Anaise, D., and Rapaport, F.T. Specificity of immune complex/complement deposits in the mediation of immunologic injury to renal allografts. Transpl. Proc., 21:278, 1989.
82. Waltzer, W.C., Shabtai, M., Anaise, D., and Rapaport, F.T. Usefulness and
limitations of Doppler ultrasonography in the evaluation of post -operative renal allograft dysfunction. Transpl. Proc., 21:1901, 1989.
83. Shabtai, M., Waltzer, W.C., Anaise, D., Miller, F., and Rapaport, F.T. Implication of IgA and complement in the alterations in renal blood flow associated with allograft rejection. Transpl. Proc., 21:352, 1989.
84. Shabtai, M., Anaise, D., Miller, F., Oster, Z.H., Atkins, H., Waltzer, W.C., Yland, M.J., and Rapaport, F.T. The predictive value of renal cortical perfusion indices during acute allograft rejection crises. Transpl. Proc., 21:1899, 1989.
85. Anaise, D., Yland, M.J., Ishimaru, M., Shabtai, M., Hurley, S., Waltzer, W.C., and Rapaport, F.T. Organ procurement from non heart-beating cadaver donors. Transpl. Proc., 21:1211, 1989.
86. Shabtai, M., Anaise, D., Frei, L., Waltzer, W.C., Frischer, Z., Jao, S., Miller, F., and Rapaport, F.T. Malakoplakia in renal transplantation - an expression of altered tissue reactivity under immunosuppression. Transpl. Proc., 1989, Aug;21(4):3725-7
87. Shabtai, M., Miller, F., Lane, B., Waltzer, W.C., Anaise, D., Arbeit, L., and
Rapaport, F.T. Nephrotic syndrome following renal transplantation. Transpl. Proc., 1989, Aug; 21(4):3733-7
88. Shabtai, M., Waltzer, W.C., Shabtai, E., Anaise, D., Miller, F. and Rapaport, F.T. Multivariate and Boolean factor analysis of immune complex /complement deposits and their effect on renal blood flow during

allograft rejection. Abstracts of the 84th Annual Convention of the American Urological Association, Dallas, Texas, May 7-11, 1989.
89. Waltzer, W.C., Pullis, C., Shabtai, M., Khoo, N., Anaise, D. and Rapaport, F.T. Peripheral blood natural killer (NK) cells in acute renal allograft recipients. The FASEB J., 3:A1235, 1989.
90. Shabtai, M., Pullis, C., Waltzer, W.C., Khoo, N., Anaise, D. and Rapaport, F.T. T-cell activation markers in acute renal allograft rejection. The FASEB J., 3:A1235, 1989.
91. Anaise, D., Madariaga, J., Gonda, A., Ishimaru, M., Anderson, E., Shabtai, M., Waltzer, W.C. and Rapaport, F.T. Protective effects of a calmodulin inhibitor on the microcirculation of cold stored livers. The FASEB J., 3:A600, 1989.
92. Anaise, D., Ishimaru, M., Madariaga, A., Irisawa, A Lane, B., Sonoda, K., Zeidan B, Shabtai M, and Rapaport, F.T. Protective effects of trifluoperazine on the microcirculation of cold stored livers. Transpl., vol 50, 6, 933 1990
93. Anaise, D., Smith, Fr. R., Ishimaru, M., Waltzer, W.C., Shabtai, M., Hurley, S. and Rapaport, F.T. An approach to organ salvage from non-heartbeating cadaver donors under existing legal and ethical requirements for transplantation. - Transplantation 1990 Feb;49(2):290-4
94. Waltzer, W.C., Smith, Fr. R., Anaise, D. and Rapaport, F.T. Equity in organ
distribution: A plea for a return to reality. Transl. Proc., Transplant Proc 1989 Jun;21(3):3388-9; discussion 3413-8
95. Anaise, D., Shabtai, E., Shabtai, M., Ishimaru, M., Irisawa, A., Bowmann, B A., Waltzer, W.C. and Rapaport, F.T. Objective numerical criteria for measurement of the severity of delayed graft function produced by different organ procurement and preservation techniques in renal transplantation. - Transplant Proc 1990 Apr;22(2):392-3
96. Shabtai M Walter WC Frischer Z Khoo NT Anaise D Rapaport FT TI - Rectus muscle flap for repair of refractory bladder fistula following renal transplantation: a case report - J Urol 1990 Feb;143(2):354-5
97. Shabtai M - Waltzer WC - Shabtai E - Anaise D - Frischer Z - Miller F – Rapaport FT - Multivariate and Boolean factor analysis of immune complex/complement deposits and their effects on renal blood flow during allograft rejection. - J Urol 1990 Feb;143(2):237-8
98. Rapaport FT - Anaise D - Organ donation-1990. - Transplant Proc 1991 Feb;23(l Pt 2):899-900
99. Shabtai M - Anaise D - Shabtai E - Raisbeck AP - Malinowski K - Oster Z -
Atkins H - Waltzer WC - Rapaport FT Renal blood flow in the immediate post-transplant period as an index of the efficacy of organ procurement and
preservation. Transplant Proc 1990 Oct;22(5):2366-8

100. Rapaport FT Waltzer WC - Anaise D - How can one balance duty to all cultures and ethnic groups with effective procurement Transplant Proc 1990 Jun;22(3):1007-9
101. Shabtai M Waltzer WC Anaise D Shabtai EL Rapaport FT Relevance of the "center effect" to the utilization of scarce resources for renal transplantation. Transplant Proc (1991 Apr) 23(2):1882-5
102. Yland MJ Anaise D Ishimaru M Rapaport FT New pulsatile perfusion method for non-heart-beating cadaveric donor organs: a preliminary report.
Transplant Proc (I 993 Dec) 25(6):3087-90
103. Anaise D Rapaport FT Use of non-heart-beating cadaver donors in clinical
organ transplantation-logistics, ethics, and legal considerations. Transplant Proc (1993 Feb) 25(1 Pt 2):1507-8
104. Rapaport FT Anaise D Technical aspects of organ procurement from the non-heart-beating cadaver donor for clinical transplantation. Transplant Proc (1993 Apr) 25(2):2153-5
105. Mozes Nff Venkat KK Kupin W Dumler F Gracida C Uniewski M Anaise D Tang DH Is the routine use of induction immunosuppression with ALG or OKT3 justified in cadaveric renal transplantation? Transplant Proc (1993 Feb) 25(1 Pt l):575-6
106. Kupin W Venkat KK Ikerniyashiro D Ocdol H Mozes M Anaise D Johnson C Morbidity of intraoperative OKT3 administration in primary eadaveric renal transplant recipients. Transplant Proc (1993 Feb) 25

Made in the USA
Lexington, KY
18 May 2018